Comparative Effectiveness Review
Number 115

Childhood Obesity Prevention Programs: Comparative Effectiveness Review and Meta-Analysis

Prepared for:
Agency for Healthcare Research and Quality
U.S. Department of Health and Human Services
540 Gaither Road
Rockville, MD 20850
www.ahrq.gov

Contract No. 290-2007-10061-I

Prepared by:
Johns Hopkins University Evidence-based Practice Center
Baltimore, MD

Investigators:
Youfa Wang, M.D., Ph.D.
Yang Wu, M.S.
Renee F. Wilson, M.S.
Sara Bleich, Ph.D.
Larry Cheskin, M.D.
Christine Weston, Ph.D.
Nakiya Showell, M.D., M.P.H.
Oluwakemi Fawole, M.D., M.P.H.
Brandyn Lau, M.P.H.
Jodi Segal, M.D., M.P.H.

AHRQ Publication No. 13-EHC081-EF
June 2013

This report is based on research conducted by the Johns Hopkins University Evidence-based Practice Center (EPC) under contract to the Agency for Healthcare Research and Quality (AHRQ), Rockville, MD (Contract No. 290-2007-10061-I). The findings and conclusions in this document are those of the authors, who are responsible for its contents; the findings and conclusions do not necessarily represent the views of AHRQ. Therefore, no statement in this report should be construed as an official position of AHRQ or of the U.S. Department of Health and Human Services.

The information in this report is intended to help health care decisionmakers—patients and clinicians, health system leaders, and policymakers, among others—make well-informed decisions and thereby improve the quality of health care services. This report is not intended to be a substitute for the application of clinical judgment. Anyone who makes decisions concerning the provision of clinical care should consider this report in the same way as any medical reference and in conjunction with all other pertinent information, i.e., in the context of available resources and circumstances presented by individual patients.

This report may be used, in whole or in part, as the basis for development of clinical practice guidelines and other quality enhancement tools, or as a basis for reimbursement and coverage policies. AHRQ or U.S. Department of Health and Human Services endorsement of such derivative products may not be stated or implied.

This document is in the public domain and may be used and reprinted without special permission. Citation of the source is appreciated.

Persons using assistive technology may not be able to fully access information in this report. For assistance contact EffectiveHealthCare@ahrq.hhs.gov.

Suggested citation: Wang Y, Wu Y, Wilson RF, Bleich S, Cheskin L, Weston C, Showell N, Fawole O, Lau B, Segal J. Childhood Obesity Prevention Programs: Comparative Effectiveness Review and Meta-Analysis. Comparative Effectiveness Review No. 115. (Prepared by the Johns Hopkins University Evidence-based Practice Center under Contract No. 290-2007-10061-I.) AHRQ Publication No. 13-EHC081-EF. Rockville, MD: Agency for Healthcare Research and Quality; June 2013. www.effectivehealthcare.ahrq.gov/reports/final.cfm.

Preface

The Agency for Healthcare Research and Quality (AHRQ), through its Evidence-based Practice Centers (EPCs), sponsors the development of systematic reviews to assist public- and private-sector organizations in their efforts to improve the quality of health care in the United States. These reviews provide comprehensive, science-based information on common, costly medical conditions, and new health care technologies and strategies.

Systematic reviews are the building blocks underlying evidence-based practice; they focus attention on the strength and limits of evidence from research studies about the effectiveness and safety of a clinical intervention. In the context of developing recommendations for practice, systematic reviews can help clarify whether assertions about the value of the intervention are based on strong evidence from clinical studies. For more information about AHRQ EPC systematic reviews, see www.effectivehealthcare.ahrq.gov/reference/purpose.cfm.

AHRQ expects that these systematic reviews will be helpful to health plans, providers, purchasers, government programs, and the health care system as a whole. Transparency and stakeholder input are essential to the Effective Health Care Program. Please visit the Web site (www.effectivehealthcare.ahrq.gov) to see draft research questions and reports or to join an email list to learn about new program products and opportunities for input.

We welcome comments on this systematic review. They may be sent by mail to the Task Order Officer named below at: Agency for Healthcare Research and Quality, 540 Gaither Road, Rockville, MD 20850, or by email to epc@ahrq.hhs.gov.

Carolyn M. Clancy, M.D.
Director
Agency for Healthcare Research and Quality

Jean Slutsky, P.A., M.S.P.H.
Director, Center for Outcomes and Evidence
Agency for Healthcare Research and Quality

Stephanie Chang, M.D., M.P.H.
Director, EPC Program
Center for Outcomes and Evidence
Agency for Healthcare Research and Quality

Christine Chang, M.D., M.P.H.
Task Order Officer
Center for Outcomes and Evidence
Agency for Healthcare Research and Quality

Acknowledgments

The authors gratefully acknowledge the following individuals for their contributions to this project: Allen Zhang, B.S., Melissa McPheeters, M.P.H., Ph.D., Christine Chang, M.D., M.P.H., Dorothy T. Chiu, M.S.P.H., Eric Vohr, M.A., Xiaoli Chen, M.D., Jung Won Min, Ph.D., Tuan T. Nguyen, M.D., Ph.D., and Cai Li, M.D.

Key Informants

In designing the study questions, the EPC consulted several Key Informants who represent the end-users of research. The EPC sought the Key Informant input on the priority areas for research and synthesis. Key Informants are not involved in the analysis of the evidence or the writing of the report. Therefore, in the end, study questions, design, methodological approaches, and/or conclusions do not necessarily represent the views of individual Key Informants.

Key Informants must disclose any financial conflicts of interest greater than $10,000 and any other relevant business or professional conflicts of interest. Because of their role as end-users, individuals with potential conflicts may be retained. The TOO and the EPC work to balance, manage, or mitigate any conflicts of interest.

The list of Key Informants who participated in developing this report follows:

Benjamin Caballero, M.D., Ph.D.
Johns Hopkins University
School of Public Health
Baltimore, MD

Jean-Pierre Chanione, M.D., Ph.D.
Department of Pediatrics
University of British Columbia
Vancouver, BC, Canada

Cheryl DePinto, M.D., M.P.H.
Department of Health and Mental Hygiene
Baltimore, MD

William Dietz, M.D., Ph.D.
Director of the Division of Nutrition,
   Physical Activity, and Obesity
Centers for Disease Control and Prevention
Atlanta, GA

Allison Field, Sc.D.
Harvard University
Department of Pediatrics
Boston, MA

Stacey Passaro, M.Eng.
Passaro Engineering
Baltimore, MD

Joanne Spahn, M.S., R.D.
Nutrition Evidence Analysis Library
U.S. Department of Agriculture
Washington, DC

Technical Expert Panel

In designing the study questions and methodology at the outset of this report, the EPC consulted several technical and content experts. Broad expertise and perspectives were sought. Divergent and conflicted opinions are common and perceived as healthy scientific discourse that results in a thoughtful, relevant systematic review. Therefore, in the end, study questions, design, methodologic approaches, and/or conclusions do not necessarily represent the views of individual technical and content experts.

Technical Experts must disclose any financial conflicts of interest greater than $10,000 and any other relevant business or professional conflicts of interest. Because of their unique clinical or content expertise, individuals with potential conflicts may be retained. The TOO and the EPC work to balance, manage, or mitigate any potential conflicts of interest identified.

The list of Technical Experts who participated in developing this report follows:

Benjamin Caballero, M.D., Ph.D.
Johns Hopkins University
School of Public Health
Baltimore, MD

William Dietz, M.D., Ph.D.
Director of the Division of Nutrition,
  Physical Activity, and Obesity
Centers for Disease Control and Prevention
Atlanta, GA

Shiriki Kumanyika, Ph.D., M.P.H.
University of Pennsylvania
School of Medicine
Philadelphia, PA

Anne Scheimann, M.D., M.B.A.
Johns Hopkins University
School of Medicine
Baltimore, MD

Joanne Spahn, M.S., R.D.
Nutrition Evidence Analysis Library
U.S. Department of Agriculture
Washington, DC

Susan Yanovski, M.D.
National Institute of Diabetes and Digestive
  and Kidney Disorders
Bethesda, MD

Peer Reviewers

Prior to publication of the final evidence report, EPCs sought input from independent Peer Reviewers without financial conflicts of interest. However, the conclusions and synthesis of the scientific literature presented in this report does not necessarily represent the views of individual reviewers.

Peer Reviewers must disclose any financial conflicts of interest greater than $10,000 and any other relevant business or professional conflicts of interest. Because of their unique clinical or content expertise, individuals with potential nonfinancial conflicts may be retained. The TOO and the EPC work to balance, manage, or mitigate any potential nonfinancial conflicts of interest identified.

The list of Peer Reviewers follows:

Laurie Anderson, Ph.D., M.P.H.
Centers for Disease Control and Prevention
Scientific Information and Dissemination
  Branch
Atlanta, GA

David Katz, M.D., M.P.H.
Yale University
School of Medicine
Derby, CT

Tim Lobstein, Ph.D.
Director of Policy and Programmes
IASO – The International Association for
  the Study of Obesity
London, United Kingdom

Kristine Madsen, M.D.
University of California, San Francisco
School of Medicine
San Francisco, CA

Joshua Sharfstein, M.D.
Secretary, Maryland Department of Health
  and Mental Hygiene
Baltimore, MD

Susan Woolford, M.D., M.P.H.
University of Michigan
Department of Pediatrics and
  Communicable Diseases
Ann Arbor, MI

Childhood Obesity Prevention Programs: Comparative Effectiveness Review and Meta-Analysis

Structured Abstract

Objectives. Childhood obesity is a serious health problem in the United States and worldwide. More than 30 percent of American children and adolescents are overweight or obese. We assessed the effectiveness of childhood obesity prevention programs by reviewing all interventional studies that aimed to improve diet, physical activity, or both and that were conducted in schools, homes, primary care clinics, childcare settings, the community, or combinations of these settings in high-income countries. We also reviewed consumer health informatics interventions. We compared the effects of the interventions on weight-related outcomes (e.g., body mass index [BMI], waist circumference, percent body fat, skinfold thickness, prevalence of obesity and overweight); intermediate outcomes (e.g., diet, physical activity); and obesity-related clinical outcomes (e.g., blood pressure, blood lipids).

Data sources. We searched MEDLINE®, Embase®, PsycInfo®, CINAHL®, clinicaltrials.gov, and the Cochrane Library through August 11, 2012.

Methods. Two reviewers independently reviewed each article for eligibility. For each study, one reviewer extracted the data and a second reviewer verified the accuracy. Both reviewers assessed the risk of bias for each study. Together, the reviewers graded the strength of the evidence (SOE) supporting interventions—diet, physical activity, or both—in each setting for the outcomes of interest. We quantitatively pooled the results of studies that were sufficiently similar. Only experimental studies with followup of at least 1 year (6 months for studies in school settings) were included. We abstracted data on comparisons of intervention versus control.

Results. We identified 34,545 unique citations and included 131 articles describing 124 interventional studies. The majority of the interventions (104 studies) were school based, although many of them included components delivered in other settings. Most were conducted in the United States and in the past decade. Results of four studies were pooled for BMI and four for BMI z-score in the school-only setting; results of five school-home studies were pooled for BMI. Other studies tested interventions delivered at home (n=6), in primary care (n=1), in childcare (n=4), and in the community (n=9). Six studies tested consumer health informatics interventions. For obesity prevention, the following settings and interventions showed benefit: school-based—diet or physical activity interventions (SOE moderate); school-based with a home component—physical activity interventions (SOE high) and both diet and physical activity (SOE moderate); school-based with home and community components—diet and physical activity interventions (SOE high); school-based with a community component—diet and physical activity interventions (SOE moderate); community with a school component—diet and physical activity interventions (SOE moderate). The strength of the evidence is either low or insufficient for the remainder of the interventions and settings.

Conclusions. The evidence is moderate about the effectiveness of school-based interventions for childhood obesity prevention. Physical activity interventions in a school-based setting with a family component or diet and physical activity interventions in a school-based setting with home and community components have the most evidence for effectiveness. More research is needed to test interventions in other settings, such as those testing policy, environmental, and consumer health informatics strategies.

Contents

Tables

Figures

Appendixes

Executive Summary

Background

The epidemic of childhood obesity is threatening America's children.[1-3] Overweight children and adolescents are at greater risk for health problems compared with their normal-weight counterparts and are more likely to become obese adults.[4] Obese children and adolescents are more likely to have serious health conditions, such as cardiovascular, metabolic, and psychosocial illnesses; type 2 diabetes; hypertension; high cholesterol; stroke; heart disease; nonalcoholic fatty liver disease; certain cancers; and arthritis. Other reported health consequences of childhood obesity include eating disorders and mental health issues, such as depression and low self-esteem.

Childhood obesity is highly prevalent in the United States.[5] Data from the 2007–08 National Health and Nutrition Examination Survey indicate that 17 percent of U.S. children and adolescents (ages 2–19 years) were obese, and approximately 30 percent were either overweight or obese.[2] Some minority groups, such as African-Americans, Hispanics, and Native Americans, and low-income groups are at higher risk of obesity.[1] Obesity is the result of biological, behavioral, social, environmental, and economic factors and the complex interactions among these factors that promote a positive energy balance. At present, the way that these factors contribute to the disparities in obesity prevalence among population groups in the United States is poorly understood. Nevertheless, a growing body of research suggests that many factors interact, including individual factors, home influences, the school environment, factors in the local community, and policies implemented at the regional and national level. They can contribute to obesogenic environments and affect children's weight.[6] A number of leading health organizations and expert panels, including the World Health Organization[7] and an Institute of Medicine expert panel, have recommended comprehensive interventions to fight the growing obesity epidemic.[8,9]

For this review, we differentiate between prevention, often called "intervention" in the childhood obesity research field, and treatment, also called "weight management" or "weight loss." The main goal of most childhood obesity prevention programs is to prevent nonoverweight children from becoming overweight or obese, while the primary objective of obesity treatment programs is for pediatric patients to lose weight. Programs designed for obesity prevention may also help overweight or obese children lose or stabilize their weight. The present review focuses on prevention. A recent Agency for Healthcare Research and Quality (AHRQ) report[10] reviewed the targeted treatment of overweight or obese children, so we did not address that topic in this review.

Types of Interventions

This report focuses on childhood obesity prevention studies, which are aimed at preventing children from gaining excessive body weight and reducing their risk of developing obesity. Unlike weight-loss interventions for obese or overweight children, these interventions may not have a goal of helping children lose weight. However, prevention studies often include all children in a population, and therefore include obese and overweight children.

Interventions to prevent obesity in children largely aim to modify diet, physical activity, or sedentary activity. Because the interventions vary substantially depending on the setting, we have organized this report first by the primary setting where the interventions took place (e.g., school, home) and then by the interventions within that setting. This should facilitate use of the report, as it is expected that decisionmakers are best able to implement interventions in the settings over which they have control (e.g., schools). We focus in this report on the comparative effectiveness of interventions; thus, outcomes need to be compared between two groups, each of which received an intervention, or between two groups, one of which received usual care or no intervention.

School-Based Interventions

These interventions took place primarily in schools, although they might also have involved parents and/or community or home activities (e.g., homework, students bringing home fliers).

Home-Based Interventions

These took place in the child's home (e.g., interventions to alter the foods purchased for home use, family fitness).

Primary Care-Based Interventions

These took place in the offices of a primary care practitioner, a clinic, or other health care entity delivering primary health care to children. We classified primary care–based interventions that included a health informatics component under primary-care interventions. Note that we classified any school-based health care as a school-based intervention.

Childcare-Based Interventions

These were interventions in settings where children received nonparental/noncustodial care, generally outside the home. We classified interventions delivered in school-based aftercare programs as school-based interventions. We classified childcare interventions delivered in other settings as childcare-based interventions.

Community-Based and Environment-Level Interventions

These included interventions delivered by enforcement of policies or legislation, or by changes to the built environment. Additionally, these interventions involved interaction with the community (a group of individuals that existed prior to the intervention and that shared one or more common characteristics, such as the YMCA or church groups).[11] Note that we classified school-based policies with the school-based interventions.

Consumer Health Informatics-Based Interventions

Consumer health informatics (CHI) are technologies that deliver interventions and information indirectly (as opposed to in person) to patients or individuals in the community. These interventions might include Web-based, phone-based, and video-based programs, games, and information storehouses.

Scope of the Review

We compared the effectiveness of obesity prevention programs for children and adolescents conducted in the United States and other high-income countries.

We reviewed all studies of children that tested interventions of diet, physical activity, or any combination of these in any setting or combinations of settings (e.g., school, home, primary care, childcare, CHI) over at least 1 year, with the exception of school-based studies or studies in other settings with a school component, which required only 6 months.

We compared the effects of the interventions on outcomes related to weight or body composition (e.g., body mass index [BMI], weight, BMI-z score [measure of relative weight adjusted for age and sex], waist circumference, percent body fat, skinfold thickness, prevalence of obesity or overweight); clinical outcomes related to obesity (e.g., blood pressure, blood lipids); behavioral outcomes related to energy balance (e.g., dietary intake, physical activity, sedentary behaviors); and adverse effects of interventions (Table A and Figure A).

Key Questions

The Key Questions (KQs) are as follows:

Key Question 1. What is the comparative effectiveness of school-based interventions for the prevention of obesity or overweight in children?

Key Question 2. What is the comparative effectiveness of home-based interventions for the prevention of obesity or overweight in children?

Key Question 3. What is the comparative effectiveness of primary care–based interventions for the prevention of obesity or overweight in children?

Key Question 4. What is the comparative effectiveness of childcare setting–based interventions for the prevention of obesity or overweight in children?

Key Question 5. What is the comparative effectiveness of community-based or environment-level interventions for the prevention of obesity or overweight in children?

Key Question 6. What is the comparative effectiveness of consumer health informatics applications for the prevention of obesity or overweight in children?

Key Question 7. What is the comparative effectiveness of multisetting interventions for the prevention of obesity or overweight in children?

Table A. Characteristics of the studies according to the PICOTS framework

PICOTS Elements	Characteristics
Population(s)	All children are in the range of 2–18 years, regardless of BMI classification.

Interventions	KQ1: Diet, physical activity, or combination interventions delivered in schools
	   • Includes nutrition education, nutrition, diet, healthy eating, parenting styles, education, policy
	KQ2: Diet, physical activity, or combination interventions delivered or implemented in the home
	   • Includes healthy eating education, parenting styles, education
	KQ3: Diet, physical activity, or combination interventions delivered or recommended in a primary care setting
	   • Includes patient, parent, and family counseling; referrals to nutritionists
	KQ4: Diet, physical activity, or combination interventions delivered in a childcare setting
	   • Includes menu changes, physical activity, policy
	KQ5: Diet, physical activity, or combination interventions delivered or implemented at the community level or through environmental modification
	   • Includes physical activity, farmers' markets, community gardens, cooking lessons, policy, green space, food store accessibility, access to healthy food choices
	KQ6: Diet, physical activity, or combination interventions delivered with consumer health informatics
	   • Includes Web-based interventions, cell phone–based interventions
	KQ7: Diet, physical activity, or combination interventions delivered across a combination of settings

Comparisons	No intervention Usual care or other interventions by settings Note: We compare the intervention group vs. the control group (i.e., those who did not receive the intervention or received usual care or other interventions) within each study and then across studies within the same setting (e.g., schools, childcare centers).

Outcomes	Primary outcomes
	   • Weight-related or body composition outcomes, including BMI or BMI distribution in the population, adiposity or other weight measures, and prevalence of obesity or overweight
	Intermediate outcomes
	   • Dietary intake, fruit and vegetable intake, fatty food intake, sugar-sweetened beverage intake, physical activity, sedentary activity
	Adverse effects
	   • Eating disorders, psychosocial outcomes, impact on growth and development, injury, cost
	Obesity-related clinical outcomes
	   • Cardiovascular outcomes, metabolic outcomes

Timing	Outcome assessment must be at least 6 months from the baseline assessment for KQ1 school-based interventions. Outcome assessment must be at least 1 year from the baseline assessment for KQs 2 through 7 if it does not include school-based interventions. Outcome assessment must be at least 6 months from the baseline assessment for KQs 2 through 7 if the KQ does include school-based interventions.
Setting	Schools, home, primary care clinics, childcare settings, or community organizations; environment-level interventions; consumer health informatics; or across these settings

BMI = body mass index; KQ = Key Question; PICOTS = population(s), interventions, comparisons, outcomes, timing, and setting

Figure A. Analytic framework for comparative effectiveness of childhood obesity intervention programs

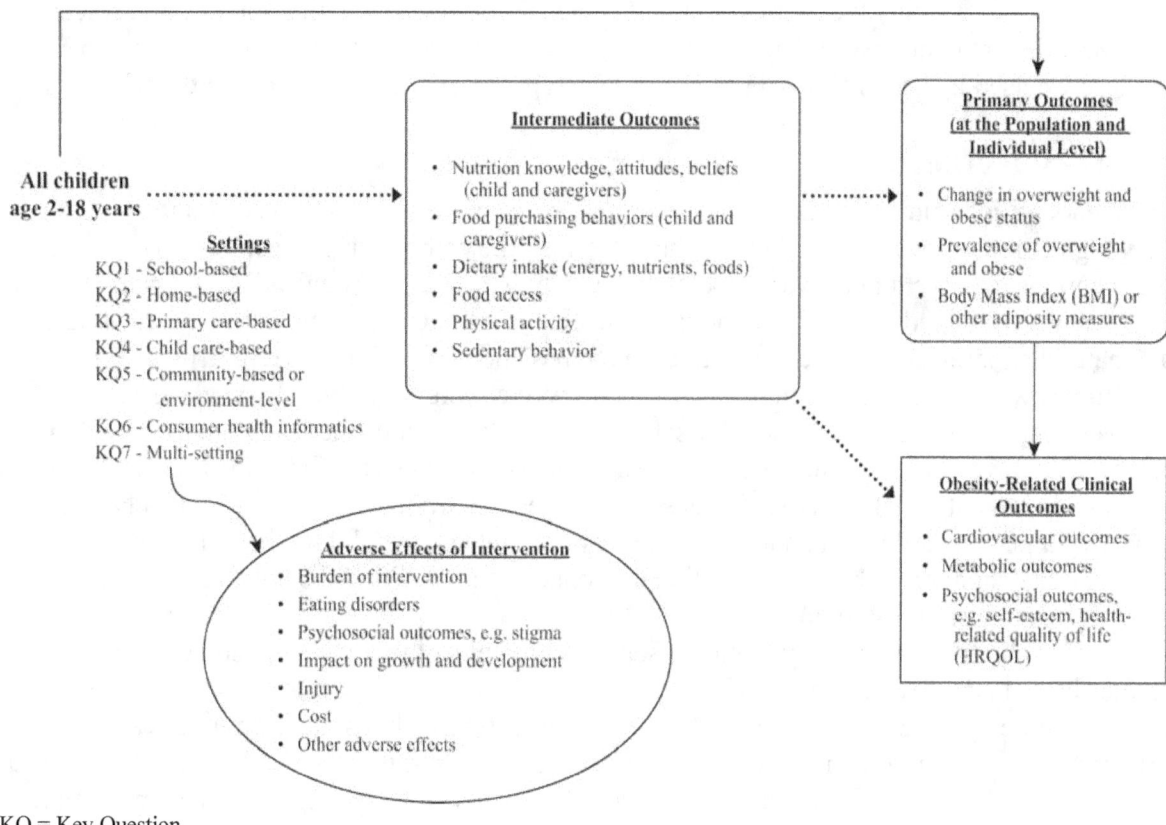

KQ = Key Question

Methods

Topic Refinement and Protocol Review

We developed the KQs with the input of a Key Informant Panel that included experts in childhood nutrition policy, academic clinicians treating obese children, representatives from public school systems, parents of obese children, representatives from professional societies focusing on nutrition and obesity, and AHRQ staff. We recruited a Technical Expert Panel that provided input to the Evidence-based Practice Center during our development of the protocol for the Comparative Effectiveness Review.

Literature Search Strategy

We searched the following databases for primary studies: MEDLINE®, Embase®, PsycInfo®, CINAHL®, and the Cochrane Library through August 11, 2012. We did not add any date limits to the search. We developed a search strategy for MEDLINE®, accessed via PubMed®, based on medical subject headings (MeSH®) terms and text words of key articles that we identified a priori. We reviewed the reference lists of all included articles, relevant review articles, and related systematic reviews to identify articles that the database searches might have missed. We uploaded the articles into DistillerSR (Evidence Partners, Ottawa, Ontario, Canada), a Web-based software package developed for systematic review and data management. We used this database to track the search results at the levels of title review, abstract review, article inclusion/exclusion, and data abstraction.

We conducted a gray literature search in ClinicalTrials.gov to identify unpublished research that was relevant to our review on July 23, 2012. The search strategies we used were comparable to those we used in the MEDLINE search, and we report them in Appendix B of the full report.

Study Selection

We identified studies conducted in the United States or other high-income countries with a very high Human Development Index[12] that described the comparative effectiveness of interventions to prevent obesity (or "excessive weight gain") in children and adolescents ages 2 to 18 years. We included only randomized controlled trials (RCTs), quasi-experimental studies, and natural experiments. (We call the latter two types "non-RCTs" in this report.)

Studies were eligible for inclusion if they followed children for at least 1 year after the intervention, or for at least 6 months for school-based intervention studies (given the length of a typical school year in the United States). We also included studies that described results from natural experiments, such as those that described outcomes from a community that had a food policy change compared with another community that did not. We did not include other observational studies, such as cross-sectional or cohort studies. We did not exclude studies based on study sample size (Table A).

Studies identified in the gray literature search had to meet the same inclusion criteria as studies identified in the regular searches.

The studies needed to compare results of an intervention with results from usual care, a different intervention, or no intervention. The interventions of interest were those that involved a modification of diet, a modification of physical activity or sedentary activity, or a combination of these. We required that the study reported on the attained differences between the intervention and control groups in weight-related outcomes, including prevalence of obesity or/and overweight, BMI or BMI distribution in the groups, and other weight and adiposity measures such as waist circumference or body fat.

We excluded studies that targeted only overweight or obese children or adolescents, and similarly excluded studies that targeted children with a chronic medical condition such as diabetes or heart disease. We excluded studies that expressly aimed to induce weight loss in the participants. We did not include studies that collected only qualitative results, such as results from interviews or focus groups. We included only articles published in English but reviewed the abstracts of non–English language articles to assess agreement with the results published in English.

Data Extraction

Two independent reviewers conducted title scans and abstract reviews, and reviewed the full articles to assess eligibility for inclusion for each study. We created standardized forms for data extraction. Each article received a double review by study investigators for data abstraction. The second reviewer confirmed the first reviewer's data abstraction for completeness and accuracy. Reviewers extracted information on study characteristics, study participants, eligibility criteria, interventions, outcome measures, the method of ascertainment, and the outcomes, including measures of variability where available.

In data extraction, we focused on primary outcomes, including BMI and related measures, such as BMI z-score and percentile, waist circumference, percent body fat, skinfold thickness, prevalence of obesity and overweight, dietary intake, physical activity, and obesity-related clinical outcomes (e.g., blood pressure and blood lipids). We also extracted behavioral outcomes that we considered to be intermediate outcomes.

Data extraction was similar for the studies we identified during the gray literature search.

Quality (Risk-of-Bias) Assessment of Individual Studies

We used the Downs and Black instrument to assess the risk of bias in the included studies.[13] We categorized the studies as having low, moderate, or high risk of bias. We rated a study as having low risk of bias only when the researchers had done all of the following: stated the objective clearly, described the main outcomes, described the characteristics of the enrolled subjects, described the intervention clearly, described the main findings, randomized the subjects to the intervention group, and concealed the intervention assignment until recruitment was complete. Additionally, the study had to have at least partially described the distributions of potential principal confounders in each treatment group. If one of the above items was not completed or if this was difficult to verify, we considered the study to have at least a moderate risk of bias. If two or more of the above items definitively were not done, we considered the study to have a high risk of bias.

Data Synthesis

For each KQ, we created a set of detailed evidence tables containing all information abstracted from eligible studies. We organized the results for each KQ by grouping the studies first according to the combination of settings where the intervention took place (e.g., a school setting along with a home setting) and then by intervention. We eliminated KQ7 in our reporting of the results because we reported on these multisetting interventions within KQs 1 through 6. Note that we reported the detailed findings of studies that examined CHI for KQ6 under other KQs. Only a summary was provided under KQ6.

We described the interventions based on their focus: (a) the targeted behavior outcomes (e.g., dietary intake or physical activity, sedentary behaviors such as recreational screentime [the time spent in front of an electronic device, including television, video games, email], or both diet and physical activity) and (b) the modality the study used to deliver the intervention (e.g., education, a modification of the environment, or instruction in self-management techniques). We reviewed the studies for outcomes for key subgroups, including outcomes reported by sex, age, or racial group, and reported the results separately by subgroups.

When we had three or more studies that had similar interventions and reported outcomes in comparable settings that were homogeneous, we pooled the primary outcomes (i.e., BMI-related measures) quantitatively (i.e., meta-analysis). We calculated pooled mean differences using a DerSimonian and Laird random-effects model.[14] We could not conduct the analysis for other outcomes due to the lack of enough comparable studies. We conducted all meta-analyses using Stata (Intercooled, version 11, StataCorp, College Station, TX). The results of each meta-analysis contributed to our assessment of the precision of the estimate of the outcome, which we used in grading the strength of evidence. We also assessed the precision of the estimate of the outcome when we could not conduct meta-analysis and used it in grading the strength of evidence.

Strength of the Body of Evidence

In our results, we reported both the strength of evidence and the magnitude of effect (e.g., the difference in changes in BMI between the intervention and control group), but strength of evidence was the primary focus. Our meta-analysis reported magnitude of effect.

We graded the quantity, quality, and consistency of the best available evidence addressing each of our KQs by adapting an evidence-grading scheme recommended in the AHRQ "Methods Guide for Effectiveness and Comparative Effectiveness Reviews" (Methods Guide).[15] We assigned grades for all weight-related outcomes by setting up a hierarchy of outcomes. Within this hierarchy, each study contributed only one weight-related measure to the grade. The hierarchy is as follows: BMI z-score, BMI, prevalence of obesity and overweight, percent body fat, waist circumference, skinfold thickness. For example, if a study measured BMI z-score and body fat, we graded only BMI z-score. We chose to use this hierarchy because these outcomes are closely correlated and encompass the scope of work. We chose six categories of intermediate outcomes: energy intake (i.e., calories), fruit and vegetable intake, fatty food intake, sugar-sweetened beverage intake, physical activity, and sedentary activity. We did not grade adverse events or clinical outcomes. We considered the four recommended domains: risk of bias, directness of the evidence, consistency across studies, and precision of the pooled estimate or the individual study estimates. We found that few studies reported precision.

We classified evidence pertaining to the KQs into four categories: (1) "high" grade, indicating high confidence that the evidence reflects the true effect, and further research is very unlikely to change our confidence in the estimate of the effect; (2) "moderate" grade, indicating moderate confidence that the evidence reflects the true effect, and further research may change our confidence in the estimate of the effect and may change the estimate; (3) "low" grade, indicating low confidence that the evidence reflects the true effect, and further research is likely to change our confidence in the estimate of the effect and is likely to change the estimate; and (4) "insufficient" grade, indicating that evidence is unavailable, there was only one study and it had moderate to high risk of bias, or a conclusion could not be drawn based on the data. We caution that a high strength-of-evidence grade is not necessarily an indicator of effectiveness; there can be strong evidence that an intervention is ineffective or even strong evidence of no effect.

We applied a grading algorithm to the body of evidence in order to have consistent grading across questions. We discussed the grades with the full group of investigators. We assessed risk of bias as described above. If the majority of studies for a given setting and comparison had the same risk of bias (low, moderate, or high), this was the risk category we assigned to that group.

We considered the body of evidence consistent in direction if 70 percent or more of the studies had an effect in the same direction (i.e., showed desirable effect vs. no desirable effect). We did not require a minimum number of studies to apply this rule; for example, a body of evidence with two positive and one negative study would be graded as inconsistent. We identified all studies as providing direct evidence, since all of the studied interventions would directly affect one of our primary outcomes. We considered a study precise if the results for the given outcome were significant at a p value less than 0.05 or had narrow confidence intervals that excluded the null. If 70 percent or more of the studies that reported statistical significance had significant results, we considered the body of evidence precise. We did not require a minimum number of studies to apply this rule; for example, a body of evidence with two precise and one imprecise study would be graded as imprecise although we recognize that, if the studies had been amenable to pooling, the precision might have increased with pooling.

Applicability

We assessed applicability (called "interpretability" in this report) separately for each question. We were guided by the PICOTS (populations, interventions, comparisons, outcomes, timing, and setting) framework, recommended in the Methods Guide.[16] We assessed whether there were features of the individual studies that limited the applicability of the study's findings, including whether the intensity of the intervention was such that it was unlikely to be widely implemented or whether the study subjects were atypical in some way.

Results

Results of the Literature Search

The literature search identified 34,545 unique citations. We excluded 28,344 citations during title screening and excluded an additional 5,600 during abstract screening. During article screening, we excluded an additional 470 articles that did not meet one or more of the inclusion criteria. We included 124 interventional studies described in 131 articles (Figure B). (Some studies were described in multiple articles.) Our gray literature search of ClinicalTrials.gov identified 3,186 potentially relevant titles. A title screen excluded 2,826 trials. Of the 342 potentially relevant trials, none met our inclusion criteria.

In total, 104 studies assessed school-based interventions, which might include other settings (KQ1). Six studies addressed home-based interventions (KQ2); one study addressed primary care–based interventions (KQ3); four studies addressed childcare-based interventions (KQ4); and nine studies addressed community-based interventions (KQ5). Several studies addressed CHI interventions (KQ6), but we describe them under other KQs. Most (83) of the 124 studies were RCTs: 69 trials for KQ1, 6 for KQ2, none for KQ3, 3 for KQ4, and 5 for KQ5. Six studies addressed KQ6.

We describe the following weight-related outcomes: BMI, BMI z-score, prevalence of obesity and overweight, waist circumference, skinfold thickness, percent body fat, and adverse events. In the full report, we also describe clinical outcomes (e.g., blood pressure, blood lipids) and intermediate behavioral outcomes (e.g., dietary intake, physical activity).

Key Question 1. What is the comparative effectiveness of school-based interventions for the prevention of obesity or overweight in children?

We describe here the large body of evidence about interventions that occurred entirely in schools and the other large body of evidence regarding interventions that occurred predominantly in schools but required the child's commitment to activities at home. Additionally, in the full report we describe interventions that occurred in the school but required involvement of the community or informatics support.

School Based Only

The strength of evidence is moderate that school-based diet or physical activity interventions prevent obesity or overweight in children. The strength of evidence is low that school-based combination diet and physical activity interventions prevent obesity or overweight in children (Table B, Appendix F).

Two RCTs, described in three articles, evaluated the effects of diet interventions on weight-related outcomes and showed a decrease in BMI or BMI z-score measures over a period of at least 1 year. These studies were specifically designed to prevent weight gain, and focused on promoting a healthy diet and reducing the consumption of carbonated drinks.

Fifteen studies reported on the effects of physical activity interventions in school on weight-related outcomes. Physical activity interventions had an impact on BMI, waist circumference in girls, skinfold thickness at 52 weeks, and percent body fat in children. These studies were designed to prevent weight gain, reducing screen-based sedentary behavior time, promoting participation in physical activity, and improving fundamental movement skills among children. One of these physical activity intervention studies that had a significant effect on percent body fat enrolled prepubertal girls, who participated in daily physical education classes led by schoolteachers. Some of the physical activity interventions also had an impact on clinical outcomes (e.g., lowering systolic blood pressure) and intermediate outcomes (e.g., increasing physical activity and reducing sedentary activities). These studies were designed to affect the cardiovascular disease risk profile and promoted daily physical activity in elementary-school children. None of these studies reported on adverse events (harms).

Thirty-seven studies assessed the effect of a combined diet and physical activity intervention on weight-related outcomes. Combination interventions show a low strength of evidence that they are effective at reducing BMI, BMI z-score, prevalence of obesity and overweight, percent body fat, waist circumference, and skinfold thickness. Studies reporting on these outcomes were designed to affect weight gain and included intensive classroom physical activity lessons led by trained teachers, moderate to vigorous physical activity sessions, nutrition education materials, and promoting and providing a healthy diet. The intervention studies with significant impact had a duration of 52 to 156 weeks. Children who followed long-term intervention programs showed significant positive changes in physical performance, whereas children in shorter studies had nonsignificant results. Similarly, the long studies had a significant effect on energy intake, reduced consumption of sweetened beverages, and increased fruit and vegetable intake.

School Based With a Home Component

The strength of the evidence is insufficient that diet interventions within school-based studies with a home component prevent obesity or overweight in children. However, the strength of evidence is high that physical activity interventions within school-based studies with a home component prevent obesity or overweight in children. The strength of evidence is moderate that combined diet and physical activity interventions within school-based studies with a home component prevent obesity or overweight in children (Table B, Appendix F).

The total number of participants in the 30 studies combined was 28,413. The mean age of participants ranged from 5.8 years to 13.2 years. Only one study tested a diet intervention alone. The more intensive of the two intervention arms showed a reduction in the prevalence of overweight and obese children. Three studies focused exclusively on physical activity interventions. All of them reported statistically significant beneficial effects of the intervention compared with the control group based on the various weight-related outcomes.

Ten (39 percent) of the 26 studies that tested diet and physical activity interventions reported a statistically significant beneficial effect (Table B). Among the 17 studies that measured BMI change, 14 showed a reduction in BMI in the intervention group relative to the control group, with the magnitude of difference ranging from -0.4 to -1.20 kg/m^2. However, only four of these changes were statistically significant.

The meta-analysis, which included four studies, was not statistically significant ($p = 0.219$). Among the seven studies that measured BMI z-score, two showed significant reductions in favor of the intervention (-0.34 and -0.38) and the rest did not.

Only one study examined and reported a significant desirable intervention effect on the prevalence of overweight and obesity (adjusted odds ratio, 0.67; 95% confidence interval, 0.47 to 0.96; $p < 0.03$). One other study found a significant difference in the prevalence of overweight (3.7%; $p < 0.05$) and obesity (2.3%; $p < 0.05$) in favor of the intervention versus the control.

Figure B. Results of the literature search

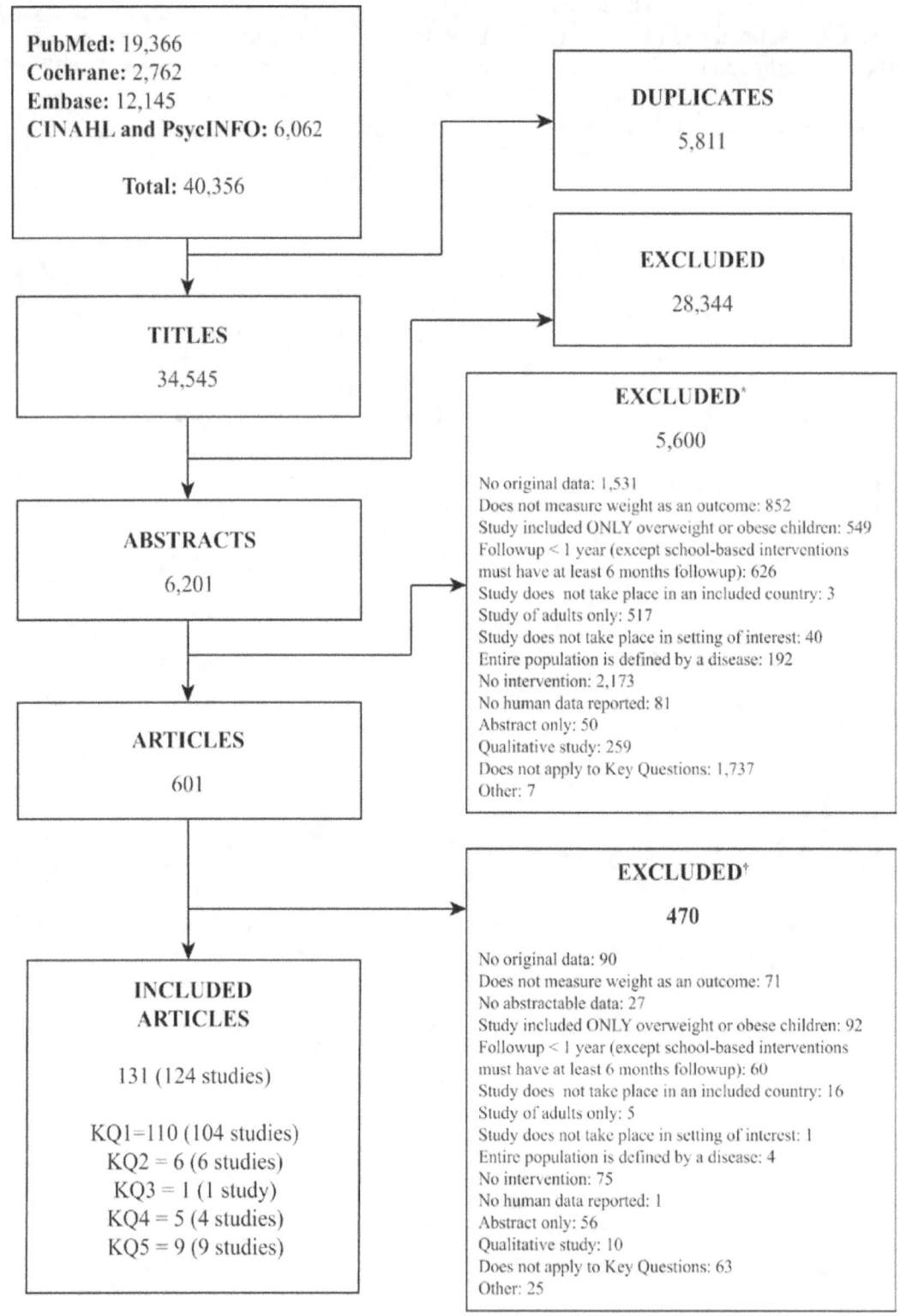

*Sum of excluded abstracts exceeds 5,600 because reviewers were not required to agree on reasons for exclusion.
†Sum of excluded abstracts exceeds 470 because reviewers were not required to agree on reasons for exclusion.

School Based With a Home and Community Component

The strength of evidence is insufficient that school-based physical activity interventions with a home and community component prevent obesity or overweight, as there was only one study and it had a moderate risk of bias. The strength of evidence is high that combined diet and physical activity interventions prevent obesity or overweight, as one study with a low risk of bias and most of the studies with a moderate risk of bias showed a favorable effect (Table B, Appendix F).

Studies on a combination of diet and physical activity interventions generally showed significant improvements in weight outcomes. Most interventions focused on education as well as structural changes to promote a healthful diet and increased physical activity. Many of the interventions did not specifically target obesity prevention.

Table B. Summary of the strength of evidence for weight-related outcomes in studies taking place in a school setting

Setting	Intervention Type, Number	Number of Enrolled Participants	Number of Studies With L/M/H RoB	RoB	Consistency	Precision	Directness	SOE
School[a]	D, 2	1,782	0/2/0	Moderate	Consistent	Imprecise	Direct	Moderate
	PA, 15	10,086	0/13/2	Moderate	Consistent	Imprecise	Direct	Moderate
	C, 37	41,875	2/27/8	Low	Inconsistent	Imprecise	Direct	Insufficient
School-home	D, 1	1,321	0/1/0	Moderate	NA	Precise	Direct	Insufficient
	PA, 3	1,654	1/2/0	Moderate	Consistent	Precise	Direct	High
	C, 26	25,438	2/20/4	Moderate	Consistent	Precise	Direct	Moderate
School-home-community	PA, 1	2,829	0/1/0	Moderate	NA	Precise	Direct	Insufficient
	C, 8	11,525	1/4/3	Moderate	Consistent	Imprecise	Direct	High
School-community	D, 1	2,950	0/1/0	Moderate	NA	Precise	Direct	Insufficient
	PA, 1	1,721	0/0/1	High	NA	Imprecise	Direct	Insufficient
	C, 4	3,017	0/2/2	Moderate	Consistent	Imprecise	Direct	Moderate
School-CHI	PA, 2	1,335	0/2/0	Moderate	Inconsistent	Imprecise	Direct	Insufficient
	C, 2	1,896	0/2/0	Moderate	Inconsistent	Imprecise	Direct	Insufficient
School-home-CHI	C, 1	589	0/0/1	High	NA	Imprecise	Direct	Insufficient

C = combination of diet and physical activity interventions; CHI = consumer health informatics; D = diet intervention; H = high; L = low; M = medium; NA = not applicable; PA = physical activity intervention; RoB = risk of bias; SOE = strength of evidence
[a] Total = 54. One study reported on diet, physical activity, and combination interventions; therefore, it was counted more than once.

School Based With a Community Component

The strength of evidence is insufficient that a diet approach or an approach combining physical activity with self-management can impact weight outcomes in a community and school setting, as only one study was included for each approach. The strength of evidence is moderate that diet with physical activity impacts BMI or BMI z-score in a community and school setting, as two of the four studies with moderate risk of bias showed a favorable effect.

Out of six studies, the one study on diet intervention showed significant improvements in BMI and prevalence of overweight and obesity.[17] It specifically targeted weight gain prevention.

The intervention focused on education as well as making structural changes to promote active physical activity. Reasons for the significant desirable effect on weight outcomes might be that the intervention specifically targeted weight gain prevention and that the sample size was large (2,950 participants).

One study reported on a physical activity intervention among girls and showed no (or nonsignificant) improvements in weight outcomes over 3 years. The intervention focused on education as well as structural changes to promote healthy diets.

Four studies on a combination of diet with physical activity interventions generally showed nonsignificant improvements in weight outcomes over a period of at least 6 months. The majority of these studies specifically targeted weight gain prevention. The focus of the interventions varied greatly—education, structural changes to promote diet changes and physical activity, or both. One reason for the nonsignificant effect on weight outcomes might have been that the sample sizes were small.

School Based With a Consumer Health Informatics Component

The strength of evidence is insufficient that school-based physical activity interventions with a CHI component prevent obesity or overweight in children. We graded the body of evidence as insufficient because it lacked precision and both studies had a moderate risk of bias. The strength of evidence is insufficient that a combination of diet and physical activity interventions prevent obesity or overweight in children. We graded the body of evidence as insufficient because it lacked precision and included studies with moderate risk of bias (Table B, Appendix F).

Two studies evaluated the effect of a physical activity intervention on weight outcomes. One quasi-experimental study included only female adolescents and the other study randomized adolescents to a control or one of two intervention groups. None of the four identified studies showed a significant intervention effect on weight outcomes.

School Based With a Home and Consumer Health Informatics Component

The strength of evidence is insufficient that school, home, and CHI approaches using combined diet and physical activity interventions prevent obesity or overweight in children. We graded the body of evidence as insufficient because it comprised only a single study with high risk of bias. No studies measured adverse events (Table B, Appendix F).

The one included study did not demonstrate significant beneficial effects on weight outcomes. The use of a non-RCT design and low intervention intensity limited this study.

Key Question 2. What is the comparative effectiveness of home-based interventions for the prevention of obesity or overweight in children?

Home Based Only

The strength of evidence is low that home-based combination interventions prevent overweight or obesity in children, and there was insufficient evidence to determine the effect of diet-only intervention in the home (Table C, Appendix F).

We included four home-based intervention studies. One study reported on a diet intervention and the remaining three studies reported on combined diet and physical activity interventions. They all were RCTs. The total followup period ranged from 52 to 104 weeks. The age range of the participants was 3 to 17 years.

None of the four studies detected a statistically significant beneficial intervention effect on BMI or other weight outcomes. However, one study demonstrated a change in the percentage of children who were overweight in favor of one intervention group. One study employed a diet intervention for girls and reported no difference in BMI, fat mass, or weight at 104 weeks between the intervention and control arms. Three combined diet and physical activity intervention trials did not detect a significant beneficial intervention effect on weight outcomes.

Home Based With a School and Community Component

No conclusions can be made about the effectiveness of a combined diet and physical activity intervention in a home setting with school and community components in prevention of obesity or overweight (Table C, Appendix F). The study we identified reported no significant difference overall in BMI between the control group and a group with combined diet and physical activity intervention.

Home Based With a Primary Care and Consumer Health Informatics Component

No conclusions can be made about the effectiveness of a combined diet and physical activity intervention in a home setting with primary care and CHI components in prevention of obesity or overweight (Table C, Appendix F). In the single study we identified, there was no difference in BMI z-score between the control group and a group with combined diet and physical activity intervention. This study was small and imprecise.

Table C. Summary of the strength of evidence for weight-related outcomes in studies taking place in the home

Setting	Intervention Type, Number	Number of Enrolled Participants	Number of Studies With L/M/H RoB	RoB	Consistency	Precision	Directness	SOE
Home	D, 1	59	0/1/0	Moderate	NA	Imprecise	Direct	Insufficient
	C, 3	262	0/2/1	Moderate	Inconsistent	Imprecise	Direct	Low
Home-PC-CHI	C, 1	878	1/0/0	Low	NA	Imprecise	Direct	Insufficient
Home-school-community	C, 1	1,323	0/0/1	High	NA	Imprecise	Direct	Insufficient

C = combination of diet and physical activity interventions; CHI = consumer health informatics; D = diet intervention; H = high; L = low; M = moderate; NA = not applicable; PC = primary care; RoB = risk of bias; SOE = strength of evidence

Key Question 3. What is the comparative effectiveness of primary care– based interventions for the prevention of obesity or overweight in children?

No conclusions can be made regarding the effectiveness of a combined diet and physical activity intervention in a primary care setting on obesity or overweight prevention (Table D, Appendix F). The one study in this setting used a quasi-experimental design. The study used educational and physical environmental approaches to target improvements in clinical decision support, counseling of families and patients on behavioral goals, and overall practice and provider management over a 78-week study period. The intervention did not result in decreased prevalence of overweight or obesity.

Table D. Summary of the strength of evidence for weight-related outcomes in studies taking place in primary care

Setting	Intervention Type, Number	Number of Enrolled Participants	Number of Studies With L/M/H RoB	RoB	Consistency	Precision	Directness	SOE
Primary care	C, 1	600	0/1/0	Moderate	NA	Imprecise	Direct	Insufficient

C = combination of diet and physical activity interventions; H = high; L = low; M = moderate; NA = not applicable; RoB = risk of bias; SOE = strength of evidence

Key Question 4. What is the comparative effectiveness of childcare center–based interventions for the prevention of obesity or overweight in children?

We identified four studies that were reported in five articles. Three RCTs and one non-RCT addressed this question. The non-RCTs tested a physical activity intervention and found significant differences in BMI and percent body fat between intervention and control groups. The remaining studies evaluated the effect of combined diet and physical activity interventions. One of them showed significant differences between intervention and control groups in weight outcomes. No studies reported on adverse events.

We could not make a conclusion about the effectiveness of interventions involving physical activity alone on prevention of obesity and overweight in a childcare setting. The strength of evidence is insufficient that a physical activity intervention in a childcare setting positively affects obesity prevention. Only one study, with a high risk of bias and imprecision, addressed the effect of the intervention on weight outcome. Combined diet and physical activity interventions showed no beneficial effect on childhood obesity and overweight prevention, with a low strength of evidence based on studies with moderate risk of bias and direct, consistent, and imprecise results (Table E, Appendix F).

Table E. Summary of the strength of evidence for weight-related outcomes in studies taking place in childcare

Setting	Intervention Type, Number	Number of Enrolled Participants	Number of Studies With L/M/H RoB	RoB	Consistency	Precision	Directness	SOE
Childcare	C, 3	2,393	1/2/0	Moderate	Inconsistent	Imprecise	Direct	Low
	PA, 1	268	0/0/1	High	NA	Precise	Direct	Insufficient

C = combination of diet and physical activity interventions; H = high; L = low; M = moderate; NA = not applicable; PA = physical activity intervention; RoB = risk of bias; SOE = strength of evidence

Key Question 5. What is the comparative effectiveness of community-based or environment-level interventions for the prevention of obesity or overweight in children?

The strength of evidence that diet, physical activity, or combinations of these interventions implemented in the community prevent obesity or overweight in children is insufficient. However, the strength of evidence is moderate that a combination of diet and physical activity interventions, when implemented in the community with some school involvement, prevents obesity or overweight in children (Table F, Appendix F).

We identified nine studies reporting on community-based or environment-level interventions. Three studies took place in the community with school involvement and used a combined diet and physical activity intervention; there was moderate strength of evidence that this setting and intervention impacted childhood obesity prevention. These studies included 4,071 participants. Two were RCTs: one was conducted in the Netherlands and another in the United States. The third was a non-RCT that took place in the United States and enrolled children over 5 years old. Two of the RCTs detected a statistically significant beneficial effect of the intervention compared with the control. No studies reported on adverse events.

Table F. Summary of the strength of evidence for weight-related outcomes in studies taking place in the community

Setting	Intervention Type, Number	Number of Enrolled Participants	Number of Studies With L/M/H RoB	RoB	Consistency	Precision	Directness	SOE
Community only	PA, 1	46	0/1/0	Moderate	NA	Imprecise	Direct	Insufficient
Community-school	C, 3	2,966 and children at 24 schools[a]	0/3/0	Moderate	Consistent	Imprecise	Direct	Moderate
Community-school-home	C, 1	1,989	0/2/0	Moderate	NA	Precise	Direct	Insufficient
Community-home	C, 2	564	0/1/1	High	Consistent	Imprecise	Direct	Insufficient
Community-home-PC-CC	C, 1	43,811	0/1/0	Moderate	NA	Precise	Direct	Insufficient
Community-school-PC-CC	C, 1	NR	0/0/1	High	NA	Precise	Direct	Insufficient

C = combination of diet and physical activity interventions; CC = childcare; H = high; L = low; M = moderate; NA = not applicable; NR = not reported; PA = physical activity intervention; PC = primary care; RoB = risk of bias; SOE = strength of evidence
[a]Mean enrollment = 1,109.

Key Question 6. What is the comparative effectiveness of consumer health informatics applications for the prevention of obesity or overweight in children?

We identified six studies meeting our inclusion criteria that evaluated the effects of CHI interventions, but they are reported in other KQs according to their settings.

KQ1 included five studies with a CHI component: four in a school-based setting with a CHI component to the intervention and one in a school-based setting with a home and CHI component. Two of the school-CHI studies reported on physical activity interventions and showed no significant intervention effect on weight outcomes. Two reported on combined diet and physical activity interventions; one showed a significant intervention effect on BMI (p < 0.001), while the other failed to show an intervention effect. The study reporting on the school-home-CHI intervention used a combined diet and physical activity intervention and demonstrated no intervention effect on weight outcomes.

KQ2 included one study with a CHI component. It took place in a home-based setting with primary care and CHI components. This study used a combination diet and physical activity intervention. It showed no difference in BMI z-score between the intervention and control during followup after adjusting for baseline BMI z-score, age, and ethnicity, but it showed significant improvements in sedentary behaviors for both sexes and in active days per week among boys. Subgroup analysis for participants with BMI at or above the 95th percentile showed a desirable but insignificant intervention effect: BMI z-score was 2.08 ± 0.02 for the intervention group and 2.12 ± 0.02 for the control during followup ($p = 0.10$).The intervention did not demonstrate an overall effect on BMI z-scores.

The six CHI intervention studies identified took place only in concert with other interventions, primarily school based, but also home-based physical activity and dietary interventions. CHI interventions contributed to improvements in intermediate outcomes, particularly physical activity, but only one of these six studies, which used a school-based diet and physical activity intervention in concert with a CHI component, demonstrated a change in weight outcomes.

Discussion

Key Findings

In total, 124 interventional studies (reported in 131 articles) met our inclusion criteria. The majority (104, 84%) were school-based studies, although many of them also included interventional components implemented in other settings, such as the home or local community. A small number of studies tested interventions primarily implemented in other settings, such as at home, in primary health care, in childcare settings, or in communities.

Based on studies conducted over periods of 6 months to 6 years, the strength of evidence is high that school-based diet and physical activity interventions with a home component or school-based combination interventions with a home and community component prevent obesity or overweight. The strength of evidence is moderate that school-based interventions contribute to obesity prevention. The strength of evidence is moderate that school-based diet or physical activity interventions with either home or community components using a combination intervention contribute to obesity prevention The evidence is either low or insufficient regarding interventions in other settings due to the small number of published studies, their moderate or high risk of bias, and conflicting results across studies.

Over half of the school-based interventions reported statistically significant beneficial effects of the intervention compared with the control in at least some of the body weight–related measures, such as BMI, BMI z-score, prevalence of overweight and obesity, waist circumference, skinfold thickness, and percent body fat.This typically means a less steep increase over time in the intervention group relative to the control group. Additionally, almost all of the studies that reported results regarding intermediate outcomes detected some statistically significant desirable effects, such as increased vegetable and fruit consumption or increased physical activity. Approximately half of the studies that reported clinical outcomes reported some statistically significant desirable effects, predominantly regarding lowered blood pressure.

Applicability

The results of this review are primarily applicable to children in high-income countries. Results are not necessarily applicable to children in middle- and low-income countries where obesity is increasing. The participants were diverse across studies, with a mix of girls and boys of multiple ethnic groups; however, only a small number of studies reported outcomes by subgroups defined by sex, race, or age. Therefore, one should apply the results cautiously to subgroups of children, particularly subgroups underrepresented in these studies. This includes very young children and selected ethnic groups, as few studies addressed these populations. The results of RCTs are often better than non-RCT results. These results address obesity prevention, not treatment.

Implications for Clinical and Policy Decisionmaking

The findings of this review can help researchers, clinical and public health practitioners, and policymakers decide on appropriate intervention strategies to combat the prevailing obesity epidemic in developed countries, and they help provide insight for future research. We need more research to test interventions that are not school based and those with innovative study design and intervention approaches. The promising results suggest that school-based childhood obesity prevention programs may help fight the rise in childhood obesity. After careful review of the individual components of the successful studies, health care professionals should be able to replicate the results in new settings, which could lead to broad implementation.

Limitations

The review was limited in scope, focusing only on prevention of obesity.

There are many differences across studies in term of settings, design, sample size and characteristics, intervention approaches, primary measures used and reported to assess the intervention effects, length of followup, and statistical analysis approaches. Such variability made it challenging to make cross-comparisons.

Given that we identified so few studies outside of the school setting, we could conduct meta-analysis only for KQ1, and we could include only a small number of interventional studies in the analysis.

We stratified the findings first based on their study settings and then by the intervention (diet, physical activity, or both). However, due to the limited sample size, we could not conduct further stratifications to explore the comparative effectiveness of the specific intervention approaches (e.g., compare educational interventions to environmental changes with pooled analyses) or the specific intermediate outcomes (e.g., compare fruit and vegetable intake to total energy intake). The reported weight outcomes and statistical methods we used to evaluate the intervention effects were heterogeneous across studies. We used BMI or related measures, such as BMI z-score, BMI percentile, and prevalence of overweight and obesity based on BMI cutpoints, as the primary outcomes, but BMI has its limitations as an indirect measure of adiposity, and it is not an ideal indicator for cardiometabolic risks. In addition, studies use different BMI cutpoints to define overweight and obesity.

Another challenge was that some studies assessed the intervention effect by comparing changes in the outcomes between the intervention and control groups, some compared between-group difference in weight outcomes only at followup, some reported on odds ratios of being overweight/obese, and others reported on the between-group difference in continuous outcome measures such as BMI. This too made comparing or pooling results challenging.

For school-based studies, we reduced the requirement for length of followup to 6 months, considering the usual length of school years. However, 6 months may be too short a time to observe the intervention effect on weight outcomes. Some studies did not state that their original goals were obesity prevention but rather stated that they aimed to reduce cardiovascular risk. We included these in the review because they included diet and physical activity interventions and reported results regarding body weight-related outcomes; thus they could shed light on the effect of childhood obesity interventions. These studies may differ from those that were primarily designed to target childhood obesity prevention. We also note that studies had variable analytic approaches and that not all accounted for correlations between individual students within classrooms. We did not differentiate those studies that did or did not address this clustering.

We attempted to identify non-English studies, but none of those we reviewed met our inclusion criteria. We limited our review to studies conducted only in high-income countries, as these results are more applicable to a U.S. population.

Future Research Needs

Many questions remain unanswered. We have identified a number of evidence gaps, many of which may warrant future research.

1. Intervention Studies Conducted in Nonschool Settings

The literature is sparse on interventions that take place in settings other than schools. We need more studies that test environment- and policy-based interventions. Although environment is a critical area for obesity prevention,[9] very few studies have tested such interventions. In addition, there is scant evidence on the impact of regional or national policies on childhood obesity prevention, including agriculture policies and regulations on food retailing and distribution.[9]

Very few studies took place in clinical settings such as primary care. Primary health care providers could play an important role in childhood obesity prevention and treatment by providing healthful eating and exercise guidelines, and regularly monitoring body weight. Studies might also be designed to compare outcomes of interventions delivered in school with comparable interventions delivered at home or in other settings.

2. Innovative Study Design and Intervention Approaches

Using well-developed behavioral theories when designing interventions may help researchers increase study success. For example, only a few studies used social marketing to deliver messages on nutrition, physical activity, and health. Studies can integrate this approach with other intervention components to promote desirable lifestyle changes. In addition, CHI may provide promise for health promotion programs such as obesity prevention. However, only six studies used CHI and only one of these significantly reduced obesity risk.

3. Intervention Studies Guided by Systems Science

Obesity in children is the result of a complex mix of biological, behavioral, social, economic, and environmental factors. Thus, the effective and sustainable prevention of obesity in children may have to target many factors, which calls for a systems approach to study design, implementation, and evaluation that takes into account multiple risk factors and the complex interactions and feedback loops among them.[18] To fill in the gaps, researchers first need to understand the contexts and challenges associated with implementing prevention programs in different settings. For example, to conduct a childhood obesity prevention program in a community setting, researchers often need to work with the local community and its key stakeholders, which usually requires considerable effort and resources. Such demand may help explain the small number of intervention studies conducted in nonschool settings. Researchers should report these contextual factors to help decisionmakers get a better idea of the applicability of a specific intervention program to their own community.

4. Studies That Test the Potential Differential Effect of Interventions

We need research that generates information about important subgroups—such as populations stratified by sex, age, race/ethnicity, or socioeconomic status—to test whether different groups respond differently to the same intervention and help tailor future interventions to maximize their benefits. To allow for such analysis we may need larger studies, which will be more costly. However, they are essential to provide valuable information for disseminating successful interventions. Such studies will test whether different groups respond to the same intervention differently and can help tailor future interventions to maximize their benefits.

Most of the studies we reviewed did not report results by population subgroup. Subgroup analysis is necessary, as the effect size of a specific intervention may be small due to the heterogeneity of intervention effects among different subgroups. For example, an intervention may have worked in girls but not in boys. This may result in overall effectiveness being insignificant. We might conduct further research that includes a stratified analysis of subgroups by sex, age, race/ethnicity, or socioeconomic status. This will help test how different groups may respond to the same intervention, and help tailor future interventions to maximize their benefits. In addition, studies have found that obesity in older children is more predictive of obesity during adulthood than obesity in younger children is.[19] We need more studies to find effective prevention strategies for obesity that occurs in late childhood and adolescence.

5. Studies With High Statistical Power

We need more studies with large sample sizes and adequate length of followup. Most childhood obesity intervention programs are not intensive enough and result in only modest behavioral changes, perhaps because many factors can affect individuals' eating and physical activity.

6. Publication of Process Evaluation Results on Interventions

The publication of process evaluation results on interventions, especially those that attempt to compare multiple intervention options, should be encouraged. Such knowledge is important for translational research and dissemination. Very few of the studies we reviewed reported process evaluation, which would provide useful insights regarding why some studies might detect a desirable effect of an intervention, while others do not. We should encourage future studies to consider study design, data collection, final analysis, and publication.

7. Application of Rigorous Analytic Approaches

We need more rigorous analytic approaches to better analyze the repeated measures collected during followup, to control for confounders remaining after randomization, and to test effect modification and heterogeneity in the treatment effect. Future studies should consider process evaluation in study design, data collection, final analysis, and publication. Very few of the studies we reviewed reported process evaluation, which would provide useful insight about why some studies but not others noted desirable effects of an intervention.

8. Obesity Prevention Research on Adolescents

Obesity in adolescents has been found to be more predictive of obesity during adulthood than obesity in younger children is.[19] We need more studies to find effective prevention strategies for obesity that occurs in late childhood and adolescence. This is an important stage of life when young people are exposed to various social and environmental factors that establish lifelong habits.

Conclusions

A large number of childhood obesity intervention studies have been conducted in high-income counties over the past three decades. They predominantly took place in school settings, and mostly in the United States. Many of the school-based studies also included intervention components implemented in other settings, such as the home and community. Overall, there is moderate to high strength of evidence that diet and/or physical activity interventions that are implemented in schools help prevent weight gain or reduce the prevalence of overweight and obesity. However, the evidence on the effectiveness of interventions primarily implemented in other settings is largely low or insufficient. We need more research to test interventions conducted in settings other than schools, especially to test the impact of policy and environmental changes. We need to encourage research that tests innovative interventions that take advantage of new technologies, behavioral theories, and methodologies, including systems science.

References

1. Wang Y, Beydoun MA. The obesity epidemic in the United States--gender, age, socioeconomic, racial/ethnic, and geographic characteristics: a systematic review and meta-regression analysis. Epidemiol Rev. 2007;29:6-28. PMID: 17510091.

2. Ogden CL, Carroll MD, Flegal KM. High body mass index for age among US children and adolescents, 2003-2006. JAMA. 2008;299(20):2401-5. PMID: 18505949.

3. Wang Y, Lim H. The global childhood obesity epidemic and the association between socio-economic status and childhood obesity. Int Rev Psychiatry. 2012 June;24(3):176-88. PMID: 22724639.

4. Serdula MK, Ivery D, Coates RJ, et al. Do obese children become obese adults? A review of the literature. Prev Med. 1993;22(2):167-77. PMID: 8483856.

5. Centers for Disease Control and Prevention (CDC). Childhood Overweight and Obesity. Updated March 31, 2010. www.cdc.gov/ obesity/childhood.

6. Hampl SE, Summar MJ. 'Weighing in' on childhood obesity. Pediatr Ann. 2009 Mar;38(3). PMID: 19353903.

7. World Health Organization. Global Strategy on Diet, Physical Activity, and Health. 2013. www.who.int/dietphysicalactivity/childhood _what_can_be_done/en/index.html.

8. Koplan JP, Liverman CT, Kraak VI. Preventing childhood obesity: health in the balance: executive summary. J Am Diet Assoc. 2005;105(1):131-8. PMID: 15635359.

9. Institute of Medicine. Accelerating Progress in Obesity Prevention: Solving the Weight of the Nation. Washington, DC: National Academies Press; 2012. www.iom.edu/ Reports/2012/Accelerating-Progress-in-Obesity-Prevention.aspx.

10. Whitlock EP, O'Connor EA, Williams SB, et al. Effectiveness of weight management interventions in children: a targeted systematic review for the USPSTF. Pediatrics. 2010;125(2):e396-418. PMID: 20083531.

11. Thomson Medstat Research Brief: Childhood Obesity: Costs, Treatment Patterns, Disparities in Care and Prevalent Medical Conditions. 2006. www.medstat.com/pdfs/childhood_ obesity.pdf.

12. UNDP. Human Development Reports. Human Development Index. http://hdr.undp.org/en/statistics/hdi/. Accessed May 21, 2012.

13. Downs SH, Black N. The feasibility of creating a checklist for the assessment of the methodological quality both of randomised and non-randomised studies of health care interventions. J Epidemiol Community Health. 1998;52(6):377-84. PMID: 9764259.

14. DerSimonian R, Laird N. Meta-analysis in clinical trials. Control Clin Trials. 1986 Sep;7(3):177-88. PMID: 3802833.

15. Owens DK, Lohr KN, Atkins D, et al. AHRQ series paper 5: grading the strength of a body of evidence when comparing medical interventions--Agency for Healthcare Research and Quality and the effective health-care program. J Clin Epidemiol. 2010;63(5):513-23. PMID: 19595577.

16. Atkins D, Chang SM, Gartlehner G, et al. Assessing applicability when comparing medical interventions: AHRQ and the Effective Health Care Program. J Clin Epidemiol. 2011;64(11):1198-207. PMID: 21463926.

17. Muckelbauer R, Libuda L, Clausen K, et al. A simple dietary intervention in the school setting decreased incidence of overweight in children. Obes Facts. 2009;2(5):282-5. PMID: 20057194.

18. Institute of Medicine. Bridging the Evidence Gap in Obesity Prevention: A Framework to Inform Decision Making. Washington, DC: National Academies Press; 2010. www.iom.edu/Reports/2010/Bridging-the-Evidence-Gap-in-Obesity-Prevention-A-Framework-to-Inform-Decision-Making.aspx.

19. Goldhaber-Fiebert JD, Rubinfeld RE, Bhattacharya J, et al. The utility of childhood and adolescent obesity assessment in relation to adult health. Med Decis Making. 2013 Feb;33(2):163-75. Epub 2012 May 29. PMID: 22647830.

Introduction

Background

Condition

Childhood obesity is a serious public health problem in the United States (U.S.) and in many other countries worldwide.[1-6] Data from the 2007-2008 U.S. National Health and Nutrition Examination Survey indicated that over 30 percent of U.S. children and adolescents (ages 2-19) years are obese or overweight.[7] Obesity prevalence increased from 5 to 10.4 percent (children aged 2-5 years), 6.5 to 19.6 percent (children aged 6-11 years), and 5 to 18.1 percent (adolescents aged 12-19 years) between 1976-1980 and 2007-2008.[7,8] Some minority groups, such as African Americans, Hispanics, and Native Americans, and low-income groups are at higher risk of obesity.[3,9-11] However, the patterns are complicated, and not all low-income or minority groups are at high risk; the relationship between obesity and social-economic status has changed over time in the U.S.[3,12] Asian Americans have a lower prevalence of obesity than other ethnic groups, while higher income African American girls are more likely to be overweight than their lower income counterparts. On the contrary, there is an inverse relationship between obesity and social-economic status in white girls. However, social-economic status factors only explain a very small portion of the variations in body mass index (BMI), approximately 1 or 2 percent. Obesity is difficult to treat and prevention of childhood obesity has been identified as a key to fight the growing global obesity epidemic.

Complex Causes of Obesity

Obesity is the result of many biological, behavioral, social, environmental, and economic factors and the complex interactions between them that promote a positive energy balance. At present, how these factors contribute to the disparities in obesity prevalence between population groups in the U.S. remain poorly understood. Nevertheless, a growing body of research adds to the understanding of a socio-ecological model for childhood obesity and suggests that many factors interact, such as individual factors (e.g., genetics, nutrition knowledge and attitude, body weight image), home influences (e.g., parenting, food served at home, parental weight status), school factors (e.g., nutrition service, curriculum including physical activity, annual BMI measure), factors in the local community (e.g., food environment, crime rate), and those at the regional and national levels (e.g., built environment, economic factors such as food prices, and food assistance programs).[13] They contribute to obesogenic environments and affect children's weight. A number of leading health organizations, including the World Health Organization[14] and the Institute of Medicine,[15] have recommended comprehensive interventions to prevent childhood obesity.[16]

Measurement of Adiposity and Classification of Childhood Obesity

The public health, research and medical communities have used various measures to assess adiposity and childhood obesity, which is a challenge for researchers and other health professionals in the field as well as for researchers conduct reviews. Although studies have mostly used BMI in the classification of obesity in adults and children, it remains controversial regarding what BMI cut points are most appropriate for a specific population.[17,18] Researchers have used different sex-age specific BMI percentile cut-points in the U.S. and worldwide.[18-21] For example, in the U.S., researchers have used two cut points, 85th (for "overweight") and 95th percentiles (for "obesity"), to define the conditions in children. Must et al. published one in 1991 based on NHANES I[22] and the Centers for Disease Prevention and Control published the other based on the 2000 U.S. Center for Disease Control and Prevention growth charts and a series of datasets.[23] In general, the values of the two sets of percentiles are similar, but researchers developed them based on different data sets and growth curve fitting techniques.[22-25]

Researchers in the field have even used different terms for overweight and obesity among children. Before the mid-2000s, key health organizations including the World Health Organization and the U.S. Center for Disease Control and Prevention recommended the use of the term of "at risk of overweight" for "overweight", and "overweight" for "obesity." Some other health organizations, such as the International Obesity Taskforce, have recommended using the terms "overweight" and "obesity" the same as they do for adults, and not using the term of "at risk of overweight." These discrepancies have further complicated the interpretation of the literature.

Additionally, BMI is an indirect measure of adiposity, and thus has several limitations. For example, it cannot distinguish between muscle mass and fat mass.[19] As a result, health care professionals have increasingly used other measures for various purposes, such as percentage of body fat measured via direct measures such as dual-emission X-ray absorptiometry, waist circumference (which measures central obesity), waist-to-height ratio, skinfold thickness, and related cut points, to assess adiposity and define obesity in adults and children. The correlations between direct and indirect measures of adiposity vary across age groups, degree of obesity, and lean muscle mass. Nevertheless, overall the correlations among them are strong.[26,27]

In summary, the definition of overweight and obesity has been evolving over time, and is not clear even today. This, combined with the controversy over the way we measure adiposity, makes it complicated to synthesize the existing literature. We recognize the need for studies to demonstrate both statistical significance (p value<0.05) and biologically or clinically meaningful change (i.e., effect size) when demonstrating an effect of intervention programs. However, to our knowledge, there is no consensus in the pediatric obesity field regarding what effect size might be considered a meaningful change.

Consequences of Childhood Obesity

Childhood obesity has many intermediate- and long-term health consequences. Overweight children and adolescents are at greater risk for health problems compared to their normal weight counterparts.[1] Overweight children and adolescents are more likely to become obese adults.[28-30] Obese children and adolescents are more likely to have adverse health conditions, such as poor cardiovascular, metabolic, and psychosocial outcomes.[31] However, the link between childhood and adulthood obesity was more prominent among older children.[32] Obesity is a risk factor for many chronic conditions, including type 2 diabetes, hypertension, high cholesterol, stroke, heart disease, nonalcoholic fatty liver disease, certain cancers, and arthritis.[30,31,33,34] It is estimated that excess weight causes 70 percent of diabetes in the U.S. Obesity increases mortality as well.[33] The other reported health risks of childhood obesity include eating disorders and mental health issues, such as depression and low self-esteem.[34] Obesity also has a lot of financial consequences. Overweight and obesity and their associated health problems have a significant economic impact on the U.S. health care system.[35] Childhood obesity in the U.S. is estimated to cost $11 billion for children with private insurance and $3 billion for children on Medicaid.[36] The health care costs of an overweight or obese child are roughly 3 times or $172 higher than the average normal-weight child, as obese children are 2 to 3 times more likely to be hospitalized and are far more likely to have health disorders than non-obese children.[37,38] Further, once developed, obesity is difficult to treat (i.e., due to the "set point theory").[39] Therefore, it is important that children develop life-long healthy lifestyles to prevent obesity.

Types of Interventions for Prevention of Childhood Obesity

Interventions for the prevention of childhood obesity have a primary goal of preventing children from gaining excessive body weight, including diet, physical or sedentary activity, or a combination of these interventions. Unlike weight-loss studies, these interventions do not have a goal of helping children lose weight. However, childhood obesity prevention studies often enroll a diverse population that includes obese and overweight children.

Scope of the Review

This report focuses on the comparative effectiveness of obesity prevention programs in children conducted in high-income countries based on a variety of outcome measures of adiposity including clinical outcomes, eating and physical activity behavioral outcomes, and potential harms. We focus in this report on the comparative effectiveness of interventions; thus, outcomes need to be compared between two groups each of which received an intervention or two groups where one group received usual care or no intervention. This review mainly compares the effects of an intervention against a control. We compared obesity prevention programs to usual care, active control, and/or other obesity prevention programs. We grouped our results based on setting and intervention (e.g., school-based dietary interventions) to shed light on the effectiveness of different interventions (e.g., diet versus physical activity). However, due to the large heterogeneity across such intervention studies and the scope of our study, we could not conduct specific statistical analysis to compare them.

The review does not include treatment of overweight or obese children, which the Agency for Healthcare Research and Quality (AHRQ) recently reviewed. We reviewed studies according to the setting where the studies were conducted and our Key Questions (KQs) are as follow.

Key Questions

Key Question 1. What is the comparative effectiveness of school-based interventions for the prevention of obesity or overweight in children?

Key Question 2. What is the comparative effectiveness of home-based interventions for the prevention of obesity or overweight in children?

Key Question 3. What is the comparative effectiveness of primary care-based interventions for the prevention of obesity or overweight in children?

Key Question 4. What is the comparative effectiveness of child-care setting–based interventions for the prevention of obesity or overweight in children?

Key Question 5. What is the comparative effectiveness of community-based or environment-level interventions for the prevention of obesity or overweight in children?

Key Question 6. What is the comparative effectiveness of consumer health informatics applications for the prevention of obesity or overweight in children?

Key Question 7. What is the comparative effectiveness of multisetting interventions for the prevention of obesity or overweight in children?

Interventions and Controversy About the Topic

We differentiate between prevention, often called "intervention" in the childhood obesity research field, and treatment, also called "weight management." The main goal of most childhood obesity prevention programs is to prevent non-overweight children from becoming overweight or obese, while the primary objective of obesity treatment programs is for obese patients to achieve healthy body weight (e.g., losing weight, improving height-to-weight ratio). However obesity prevention programs may also help overweight or obese children to lose weight or stabilize their weight. This review focuses on prevention. We did not review treatment of overweight or obese children, as a recent AHRQ report already reviewed this.[40]

Interventions to prevent obesity in children included diet (called "diet intervention" in this report), physical and/or sedentary activity (called "physical activity intervention"), or a combination of these (called "diet and physical activity intervention"). Note that a very small proportion of diet and physical activity intervention studies may also address other behaviors, such as self-weight monitoring. For clarity, and given there were a small number of such studies, we chose not to separate them from those that only diet and physical and/or sedentary activity interventions.

Some interventions included changes in individuals' knowledge, attitudes and beliefs, and some included changes in the physical environment such as food provided in the school, but all of them aimed to change the energy balance by changing diet (energy intake) or physical activity (energy expenditure) or both. A growing consensus is that we need comprehensive intervention programs that involve multiple sectors in our society or that address multiple factors affecting energy balance behaviors to fight the obesity epidemic. However, studies to date have yielded mixed results.

We identified over 20 previous systematic reviews of childhood obesity prevention. Despite the many reviews (some as recent as 2011) there were few conclusions to guide decisionmaking. The majority of them focused on school-based interventions and did not include those that took place in other relevant settings, such as home, community, and primary care. Schools are the most frequent setting for interventions as they are convenient for RCTs; it is uncertain, however, if schools are the most effective setting in which to intervene. Most only focused on BMI and obesity rates outcomes, but did not examine the other important outcomes. And some systematic reviews confined their searches to evidence from a particular geographic region, such as in China, Europe, the United Kingdom, and the U.S.; and few included any quantitative pooling, which is a one key goal of systematic reviews. Additionally, many new studies have appeared since the publication of these earlier reviews.

Organization of This Report

Because the interventions vary substantially across the settings, we organized this report first by the primary setting where the interventions took place (e.g., school, home) and then by the interventions within that setting. This should facilitate use of the evidence report as it is expected that decision-makers are best able to implement interventions in the settings over which they have control (e.g. schools). This report describes 125 studies (described in 132 articles) classified by the setting or settings (e.g., school, home) where the interventions took place. Most of the studies we included in this report took place in multiple settings (e.g., both school and home), and therefore we eliminated KQ 7 in the reporting of our results, and put those studies under one of the six other KQs depending on their primary setting of intervention.

For each KQ, we present the results according to the study design (e.g., randomized controlled trials (RCTs) vs. non-RCTs) and then the intervention (e.g., dietary changes, physical or sedentary activity changes, or both (this may also address changes such as self-weight monitoring)).

We then describe the results ordered by outcomes, such as weight-related outcomes, clinical outcomes related to obesity (e.g., blood pressure, blood lipids), behavioral outcomes (e.g., dietary intake, physical activity), and adverse effects of interventions (Table 1 and Figure 1). The weight-related outcomes include weight or body composition outcomes (e.g., BMI, weight, BMI z-score, waist circumference, percent body fat, skinfold thickness, population prevalence of obesity or overweight).

Table 1. Characteristics of the studies according to the PICOTS framework

Population(s)	All Children Between the Ages of 2 and 18 Years, Regardless of BMI Classification
Interventions	KQ 1: Examples of diet, physical activity or combination interventions delivered in schools.
	• Includes: nutrition education, Nutrition, diet, healthy eating, parenting styles,education, policy
	KQ 2: Examples of diet, physical activity or combination interventions delivered or implemented in the home.
	• Includes: healthy eating education, parenting styles,education
	KQ 3: Examples of diet, physical activity or combination interventions delivered or recommended in a primary care setting.
	• Includes: patient, parent, and family counseling; referrals to nutritionists
	KQ 4: Examples of diet, physical activity or combination interventions delivered in a child-care setting.
	• Includes menu changes, physical activity, policy
	KQ 5: Examples of diet, physical activity or a combination interventions delivered or implemented at the community level or through environmental modification.
	• Includes: physical activity, farmer's markets, community gardens, cooking lessons, policy, green space, food store accessibility, access to healthy food choices
	KQ 6: Examples of diet, physical activity or a combination interventions delivered with consumer health informatics
	• Includes: Web-based interventions, cell phone-based interventions
	KQ 7: Examples of diet, physical activity or combination interventions delivered across a combination of settings.
Comparisons	No intervention
	Usual care or other interventions by settings
	NOTE: We will compare the intervention group vs the control group (i.e., those who did not receive intervention or received usual care or other interventions) within each study and then across studies within the same setting (e.g., schools, child-care centers).

Table 1. Characteristics of the studies according to the PICOTS framework (continued)

Population(s)	All Children Between the Ages of 2 and 18 Years, Regardless of BMI Classification
Outcomes	Primary outcomes • Weight-related or body composition outcomes including in BMI or BMI distribution in the population, in adiposity or other weight measures, prevalence of obesity or overweight Intermediate outcomes • Dietary intake, fruit and vegetable intake, fatty food intake, sugar-sweetened beverage intake, physical activity, sedentary activity. Adverse effects • Correlates to eating disorders, psychosocial outcomes, impact on growth and development, injury, cost Obesity-related clinical outcomes • Cardiovascular outcomes, metabolic outcomes, psychosocial outcomes
Timing	Outcome assessment must be at least 6 months from the baseline assessment for KQ 1 school-based interventions. Outcome assessment must be at least 1 year from the baseline assessment for KQs 2 through 7 (if it does not include school-based interventions). Outcome assessment must be at least 6 months from the baseline assessment for KQs 2 through 7 (if the KQ includes school-based interventions).
Setting	Schools, home, primary-care clinics, child-care settings, or community organizations, environmental-level interventions, consumer health informatics, or across these settings

KQ = Key Question, CHI = Consumer Health Informatics

Figure 1. Analytic framework for comparative effectiveness of childhood obesity intervention program

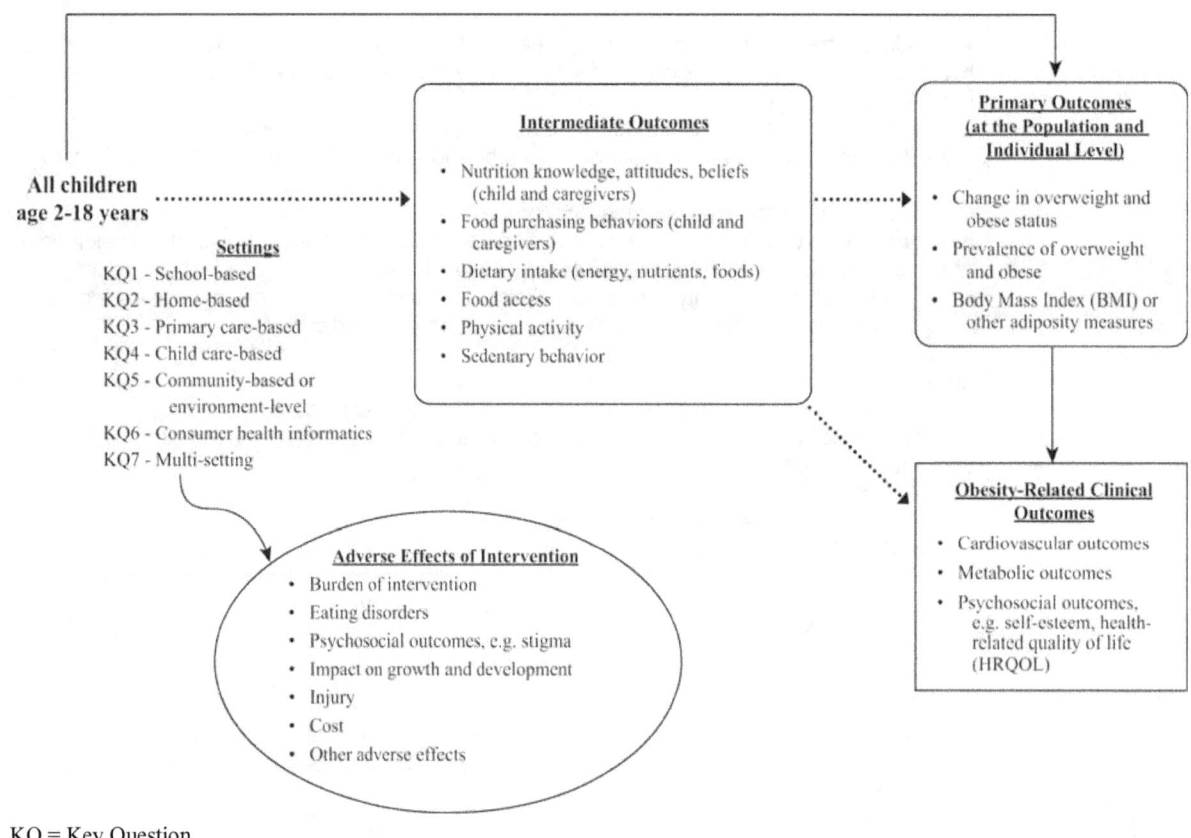

KQ = Key Question

6

Methods

The methods for this comparative effectiveness review follow the methods suggested in the Agency for Healthcare Research and Quality (AHRQ) "Methods Guide for Effectiveness and Comparative Effectiveness Reviews" (available at http://www.effectivehealthcare.ahrq.gov/ methodsguide.cfm). The main sections in this chapter reflect the elements of the protocol established for the comparative effectiveness review; certain methods map to the PRISMA checklist.[41]We determined all methods and analyses a priori.

Topic Refinement and Protocol Review

We developed the Key Questions (KQs) with the input of a key informant panel, which included experts in childhood nutrition policy, academic clinicians treating obese children, representatives from public school systems, parents of obese children, representatives from professional societies focusing on nutrition and obesity, and staff from AHRQ and the Scientific Resources Center. AHRQ posted these KQs on its Web site for public comment in July 2011 for 4 weeks and revised as needed. The KQs focus on the comparisons of methods for prevention of obesity in children. We recruited a Technical Expert Panel, which included experts on childhood obesity, primary care, obesity policy, and nutrition. These technical experts provided high-level expertise to the Evidence-based Practice Center during our development of the protocol for the comparative effectiveness review. Additionally, the Effective Health Care Program posted the KQs on its website for public comment and we discussed the KQs with the Technical Expert Panel.

Key Definitions

Obesity and Overweight

Obesity is a medical condition in which excess body fat has accumulated to the extent that it may have an adverse effect on health. For children, obesity is defined based on age-sex-specific 95th body mass index (BMI) percentiles, while overweight, based on the 85th percentile. However, different studies might have used different BMI references, for example, some studies in European countries might use the 97th BMI percentile developed based on their country-specific data for obesity. Moreover, some studies may use other measures, such as the 90th percentiles of waist circumference (to define central obesity), skinfold thickness, and percentage of body fat. Note that until recently that the WHO and the US CDC ever recommended to use the term of "at risk of overweight" for "overweight" and use "overweight" for "obesity" in children and adolescents.[19,22,23]

Interventions for Prevention of Childhood Obesity

Our team came to a consensus on the definitions of the following settings and types of interventions in order to categorize the studies that we identified in our literature search. We grouped studies by the predominant setting of the intervention as we anticipated that this would best meet the needs of the users of this report.

School-Based Interventions

School-based interventions are those studies that are carried out primarily in schools. Such interventions might also involve parents, as well some activities at home (e.g., homework, students bringing home flyers).

Home-Based Interventions

Home-based interventions are those carried out in or through the child's home. For example, these may intervene to alter the foods purchased for home use or family fitness.

Primary Care-Based Interventions

Primary-care based interventions are those carried out in or through the offices of a primary care practitioner, a clinic, or other health care entity delivering primary health care to children. Note that we classify school-based health care as a school-based intervention. Primary care-based interventions, which include a health informatics component, are classified under primary-care interventions.

Childcare-Based Interventions

Child-care settings are those where children receive non-parental/non-custodian care, generally outside the home. We classify school-based after-care programs as school-based interventions. We classify childcare interventions delivered in other settings as childcare-based interventions.

Community-Based and Environment-Level Interventions

Community-based and environment-level interventions include those interventions that result from policy, legislative, built environment, and economic/pricing/food subsidy interventions. We classified school-based policies with the school-based interventions. Additionally, these interventions involve interaction with the community (a group of individuals who exist prior to the intervention and who share one or more common characteristics such as the YMCA, Church groups).[36]

Consumer Health Informatics-Based Interventions

Consumer Health Informatics encompasses technologies focused on indirect, as opposed to face-to-face, contact with patients as the primary users of health information. This includes Web-based, phone-based, and video-based programs, games, and information storehouses.

Search Strategy

We searched the following databases for primary studies: MEDLINE® via PubMed, Embase®, PsychInfo, CINAHL®, and the Cochrane Library through August 11, 2012. We did not add any date limits to the search: PubMed catalogues articles to 1966; The Cochrane Library catalogues articles to 1989; CINAHL catalogues articles to 1982; Embase catalogues articles to 1974. We developed a search strategy for MEDLINE, accessed via PubMed®, based on medical subject headings (MeSH®) terms and text words of key articles that we identified a priori. (Appendix B) We reviewed the reference lists of all included articles, relevant review articles, and related systematic reviews to identify articles that might have been missed by the database searches. We did not request Scientific Information Packets from any manufacturers as we were not studying any pharmaceuticals or devices.

We downloaded the results of the searches and imported them into ProCite® version 5 (ISI Research Soft, Carlsbad, Calif.). We scanned for exact article duplicates; author/title duplicates, and title duplicates using the duplication check feature in ProCite. We uploaded the articles from ProCite to DistillerSR (Evidence Partners, Ottawa, Ontario, Canada), a Web-based software package developed for systematic review and data management. We used this database to track the search results at the levels of title review, abstract review, article inclusion/exclusion, and data abstraction.

We conducted a grey literature search in ClinicalTrials.gov to identify unpublished research that was relevant to our review on July 23, 2012. The search strategies we used were comparable to those used in the MEDLINE search and are in Appendix B.

Study Selection

We aimed to identify studies describing the comparative effectiveness of interventions to prevent obesity (or excessive weight gain) in children and adolescents 2 to 18 years old, conducted in the United States or other countries with a very-high Human Development Index based on the United Nations' report.[42] We included only randomized controlled trials and non-randomized trials, as we expected observational studies on this topic to be confounded and could not tested causality. We included only articles published in English, but reviewed the abstracts of non-English language articles to assess agreement with the results published in English. We did not exclude studies based on study size.

Studies were eligible for inclusion if they followed children for at least 1 year after the initiation of the intervention, or at least 6 months if it was a school-based intervention given the expectation that most studies would not observe children past the 9-month school-year (see Table 2).

The studies needed to compare results from any intervention targeting obesity prevention to results from usual care, or another different intervention, or no intervention. We also intended to include in this review studies that described results from natural experiments, such as those that described outcomes from a community that implemented a food policy change, compared to another community that did not. We did not include other observational studies, such as cross-sectional or cohort studies. We differentiated natural experiments from other observational study designs by specifying that a natural experiment was the implementation of a policy or similar intervention at a population level.

For inclusion in this review, we required that the study reported on the attained differences between the intervention and control groups in the prevalence of obesity or/and overweight, BMI or BMI distribution in the groups, or other weight and adiposity measures such as waist circumference, percentage of body fat, or skinfold thickness.

We excluded studies that targeted only at overweight or obese children or adolescents, and similarly excluded studies that targeted children on the basis of having a chronic medical condition like diabetes or heart disease. We excluded studies that expressly aimed to induce weight loss in the participants. We did not include studies that collected only qualitative results, such as from interviews or focus groups. We did not include studies published only in abstract form due to the sparseness of data in abstracts.

Trials identified in the grey literature search were required to meet the same inclusion criteria as studies identified in the regular searches.

Data Extraction

We used DistillerSR (Evidence Partners, 2010) to manage the screening and review process. We uploaded all applicable citations identified by the search strategies to the system.

Two independent reviewers conducted title scans. For a title to be eliminated at this level, both reviewers had to indicate that the study was ineligible. If the reviewers disagreed, they advanced the article to the next level, abstract review. Two investigators independently reviewed abstracts and we excluded the abstracts if both investigators agreed that they met one or more of the exclusion criteria. We tracked and resolved differences between investigators regarding abstract inclusion or exclusion through consensus adjudication. Articles promoted on the basis of abstract review received an independent parallel review to determine if we should include them in review. We resolved differences by consensus adjudication.

We created standardized forms for data extraction. (Appendix C) Each article received a double review by study investigators for data abstraction. The second reviewer confirmed the first reviewer's data abstraction for completeness and accuracy. We formed reviewer pairs that included personnel with both clinical and methodological expertise. A third reviewer audited a random sample of articles selected by the first two reviewers to ensure consistency in the abstraction of data from the articles. We did not hide reviewers from the authors, institution, or journal for each article.

Reviewers extracted information on general study characteristics, study participants, eligibility criteria, interventions, outcome measures, the method of ascertainment, and the outcomes, including measures of variability where available. We entered all information from the article review process into the DistillerSR database. We used the DistillerSR database to maintain the data, and then exported it into Microsoft Excel for the preparation of evidence tables.

Data extraction followed a similar process for the trials identified during the grey literature search. Two independent reviewers conducted title scans. For a title to be eliminated at this level, both reviewers had to indicate that the study was ineligible. If the reviewers disagreed, the article was advanced to the next level. All trials that were advanced to level 2 were screened by two reviewers and disagreements were adjudicated by a third party reviewer.

Quality (Risk of Bias) Assessment of Individual Studies

We used the Downs and Black instrument (see Appendix C) to assess the risk of bias in the included studies.[43] We opted to apply it by focusing on the questions that we felt were most relevant to this body of literature. To be considered to be a study at low risk of bias, the study must have done all of the following: stated the objective clearly, described the main outcomes, described the characteristics of the enrolled subjects, described the intervention clearly, described the main findings, randomized the subjects to the intervention group, and concealed the intervention assignment until recruitment was complete. Additionally, the study had to have at least partially described the distributions of (potential) principal confounders in each treatment group.

We categorized the studies as having low risk of bias, moderate risk of bias, or high risk of bias: (1) If we could not determine one of the above items or it was not done, we considered the study to have at least a moderate risk of being biased; (2) If studies definitively did not do two or more of the above items, we considered the study to have a high risk of bias; (3) We did not require other items that are typically expected in a well-conducted randomized trial due to the types of interventions; that is, we did not require blinding for the study to be considered a low risk of bias study, and we did not require descriptions of loss to followup and complete adverse event reporting. Studies with a high risk of bias were thought to have significant flaws that might have invalidated the results.

Data Synthesis

For each KQ, we created a set of detailed evidence tables containing all information abstracted from eligible studies. The elements that we abstracted about the interventions included the behavior (e.g., diet or/and physical activity), and the mode of delivery for the intervention (e.g., education, a modification of the environment, instruction in self-management techniques). We abstracted data on weight-related or body composition outcomes (e.g., change in prevalence of obesity, change in BMI or BMI distribution in the population, changes in adiposity or other weight measures, prevalence of obesity or overweight), obesity-related clinical outcomes, adverse effects of the interventions, and intermediate outcomes (e.g., nutrition knowledge, food purchasing behaviors, calorie intake, diet composition, physical activity). We extracted information about the primary weight outcomes at the time points of 24 weeks (for school-based studies only), 52 weeks, between 54 and 104 weeks, and greater than 104 weeks.

We pooled the outcomes quantitatively (conducted meta-analysis) when we had three or more randomized controlled trials with similar interventions in comparable settings that were homogeneous. We first confirmed that the studies were sufficiently qualitatively homogenous with respect to the population characteristics, intervention, comparison, outcomes, and timing. For studies amenable to pooling with meta-analyses, we calculated pooled mean differences using a DerSimonian and Laird random effects model.[44]We did not conduct meta-analysis regarding other measures of the intervention effects such as odds ratio or relative risk estimates due to the limited number of comparable studies that reported such results. The result of each meta-analysis contributed to our assessment of the precision of the estimate of the outcome, which we used in our grading the strength of evidence.

We identified statistical heterogeneity between the studies using a chi-squared test with a significance level of alpha less than or equal to 0.10, and an I-squared statistic with a value greater than 50 percent indicating substantial heterogeneity. We conducted all meta-analyses using STATA (Intercooled, version 11, StataCorp, College Station, Texas).

We reviewed the studies for outcomes by key subgroups including outcomes reported by sex, age, or racial group, and reported the results separately by subgroups and pooled the data where appropriate.

We describe the evidence about the following outcomes: prevention of obesity or overweight (combined outcome of all weight-related outcomes), intermediate outcomes, clinical outcomes, and adverse events. Because of the diversity of measures, we did not calculate an effect size. Furthermore, the frequent lack of reporting of measures of variation made it impossible to calculate effect sizes. Rather our conclusions indicate whether the intervention suggests benefit, no benefit, or unknown benefit. We could not explicitly state whether the reported effects met a clinically relevant threshold as this is not well established in the obesity research community.

Strength of the Body of Evidence

In our results, we reported both the strength of evidence and the magnitude of effect (e.g., the difference in changes in BMI between the intervention and control group), but strength of evidence was the primary focus. Our meta-analysis reported magnitude of effect. After synthesizing the evidence, we graded the quantity, quality, and consistency of the best available evidence addressing each of our KQs by adapting an evidence grading scheme recommended in the Methods Guide for Conducting Comparative Effectiveness Reviews.[56] In assigning evidence grades, we considered the four recommended domains including risk of bias in the included studies, directness of the evidence, consistency across studies, and precision of the pooled estimate or the individual study estimates.

We graded the evidence, for each setting, by intervention, comparator, and then by outcomes. We grouped the interventions for grading purposes as: 1) all diet interventions, 2) all physical activity interventions, and 3) all combined diet and physical activity interventions. We assigned grades for all weight-related outcomes together with each study contributing only one weight-related measure to the grade by setting up a hierarchy of outcomes. The hierarchy was set as follows: BMI z-score, BMI, prevalence of obesity and overweight, percent body fat, waist circumference, skinfold thickness. If a study measured BMI z-score and body fat, we only graded BMI z-score. We chose to use this hierarchy because these outcomes are closely correlated within an individual--particularly BMI and BMI z-score. We graded six categories of intermediate outcomes: change in energy (caloric) intake, change in fruit and vegetable intake, change in fatty food intake, change in sugar-sweetened beverage intake, change in physical activity, and change in sedentary activity. We did not grade adverse events, or clinical outcomes. Conclusions about the benefit of an intervention are unlikely to change with the addition of evidence grades for highly correlated outcomes. We did not grade adverse events, there were too few studies overall to do this. We graded selected intermediate outcomes; these were change in physical activity, change in food intake (e.g., fruit and vegetable intake, fatty foods intake, and sugar-sweetened beverage intake), change in energy intake, and change in physical activity. We chose to grade these intermediate outcomes as they are most likely to directly influence the weight outcomes.

We classified evidence pertaining to the KQs into four categories: 1) "high" grade (indicating high confidence that the evidence reflects the true effect, and further research is very unlikely to change our confidence in the estimate of the effect); 2) "moderate" grade (indicating moderate confidence that the evidence reflects the true effect, and further research may change our confidence in the estimate of the effect and may change the estimate); 3) "low" grade (indicating low confidence that the evidence reflects the true effect, and further research is likely to change our confidence in the estimate of the effect and is likely to change the estimate); and 4) "insufficient" grade (evidence is unavailable or there was only one study having more than a low risk of bias). We caution that a "high" strength of evidence grade is not necessarily an indicator of effectiveness – there can be strong evidence that an intervention is ineffective or even strong evidence of no effect.

We considered the body of evidence consistent in direction if 70 percent or more of the studies had an effect in the same direction (i.e., showed desirable effect verse not). We did not require a minimum number of studies to apply this rule, for example, a body of evidence with two positive and one negative study would be graded as inconsistent. We identified all studies as providing direct evidence since all of the studied interventions would directly affect one of our primary outcomes. We considered a study precise if the results for the given outcome were significant at a p value less than 0.05, or had narrow confidence intervals that excluded the null. If 70 percent or more of the studies that reported statistical significance had significant results, we considered the body of evidence precise. We did not require a minimum number of studies to apply this rule, for example, a body of evidence with two precise and one imprecise study would be graded as imprecise although we recognize that if the studies had been amenable to pooling, the precision might have increased with pooling.

We applied a grading algorithm to the body of evidence to have consistent grading across questions. If we found two studies with low risk of bias that had consistent direction of outcomes and no studies with a low risk of bias with outcomes in the opposite direction, we considered this to be high strength of evidence. If we found one study with low risk of bias and two or more studies with a moderate risk of bias, and they were all in a consistent direction, and no study with a low risk of bias with outcomes in the opposite direction, we considered this high strength of evidence. If there were no studies with a low risk of bias and the moderate risk of bias studies were consistent or predominantly consistent (>70 percent), we considered this moderate strength of evidence. If there were no low risk of bias studies and the studies with moderate risks of bias were inconsistent, we considered this low strength of evidence, the same is true of anything weaker than this.

Applicability

We assessed applicability separately for each question guided by the PICOTS framework as recommended in the Methods Guide for Comparative Effectiveness Reviews of Interventions.[52] We assessed whether there were features of the individual studies which limited the applicability of the study's findings to the general population.

Peer Review and Public Commentary

We invited experts in childhood obesity prevention and management, obesity policy, and individuals representing stakeholder and user communities to provide external peer review of this comparative effectiveness review. AHRQ and an associate editor also provided comments. AHRQ posted the draft report on its website for 4 weeks to elicit public comment. We addressed all reviewer comments, revised the text as appropriate, and documented our responses in a disposition of comments report that we will make available 3 months after AHRQ posts the final review on its website.

Table 2. Inclusion and exclusion criteria

Population and condition of interest	We include studies of children and adolescents aged 2-18 years, regardless of BMI classification. We exclude studies targeting only overweight or obese subjects. We exclude studies targeting subjects with diseases/chronic conditions (T2DM, CVD).
Interventions	We exclude studies that did not include an intervention aimed at obesity prevention or affecting energy-balance behaviors. We exclude studies that aim at weight loss (obesity treatment).
Comparisons of interest	Studies must compare the intervention to no intervention, usual care, or other interventions within or across settings, or compare to prior conditions for natural experiment studies.
Outcomes and timing	All studies must report changes or differences between the intervention and control groups in the prevalence of obesity and/or overweight, BMI or BMI distribution in the population, adiposity or other weight measures, such as waist circumference or body fat. Intermediate outcomes include: nutrition knowledge, attitudes, beliefs, and diet and physical activity behavior changes. Adverse effects include: eating disorders; psychosocial outcomes; Impact on growth and development; Injury; cost Obesity-related clinical outcomes include: cardiovascular outcomes; metabolic outcomes; psychosocial outcomes Outcome assessment must be at least 1-year after the baseline assessment for KQs 2 through 7 (if does not include school-based interventions). Outcome assessment must be at least 6 months after the baseline assessment for KQ 1 or for other KQ that include a school-based intervention.

Table 2. Inclusion and exclusion criteria (continued)

Type of study	We include experimental, quasi-experimental interventions and natural experiments. We exclude studies with no original data (e.g., reviews, editorials, comments). We exclude non-interventional studies (e.g., cross-sectional and cohort studies, case reports). We exclude studies published only as abstracts. We exclude qualitative studies that do not provide quantitative information on an approach of interest and weight or adiposity, such as focus groups or directed interviews We include pilot studies of an experimental design.
Setting	We include studies conducted in any of the settings described in the Key Questions. We limit our investigation to studies conducted in countries with a very-high Human Development Index.[42]

BMI = body mass index, CVD = cardiovascular disease, KQ = Key Question, T2DM = type 2 diabetes mellitus

Results

Introduction

We organized the results by Key Question (KQ) (see Introduction for a complete list of KQs). For example, if a study was primarily based in a school but had some home components, we reported the results under KQ 1 (school-based interventions). Each setting is subdivided by intervention (diet-only, physical activity-only, or combination of diet and physical activity).

Results of the Literature Search

The literature search identified 34,544 unique citations. During the title screening, we excluded 28,344 citations. During the abstract screening, we excluded 5,600 citations that met at least one of the exclusion criteria (see Chapter 2 for details). During article screening, we excluded an additional 470 articles that did not meet one or more of the inclusion criteria (see Appendix D). In total, we included 131 articles, which reported on 124 studies (i.e., some studies were described in multiple articles), in the review (Figure 2). The majority (104 out of the 124 studies) were school-based studies, which might have included intervention components conducted in other settings such as at home.

We conducted a grey literature search of ClinicalTrials.gov (see Appendix B) and identified 3,186 potentially relevant titles. A title screen excluded 2,826 of the trials. Of the 342 potentially relevant trials none that apply to this systematic review were completed, or data was not available.

Description of Types of Studies Retrieved

One hundred and four studies described in 110 articles addressed KQ 1 (school-based interventions); six studies addressed KQ 2 (home-based interventions); one study addressed KQ 3 (primary care–based interventions); four studies described in five articles addressed KQ 4 (child-care center–based interventions); nine studies addressed KQ 5 (community-based interventions); and no studies directly addressed KQ 6 (consumer health informatics–based interventions). We addressed KQ 7 (combination settings) under the above KQs.

Eighty-three studies were randomized controlled trials (RCTs). Of those, 69 addressed KQ 1, six addressed KQ 2, none addressed KQ 3, three addressed KQ 4, and five addressed KQ 5. Eighty-three studies stated that their goal was obesity prevention: 66 of these addressed KQ 1, six addressed KQ 2, one addressed KQ 3, two addressed KQ 4, and eight addressed KQ 5. Of the studies stating that their goal was obesity prevention, 54 were RCTs. Of those, 43 addressed KQ 1, five addressed KQ 2, none addressed KQ 3, two addressed KQ 4, and four addressed KQ 5.

Figure 2. Results of the literature search

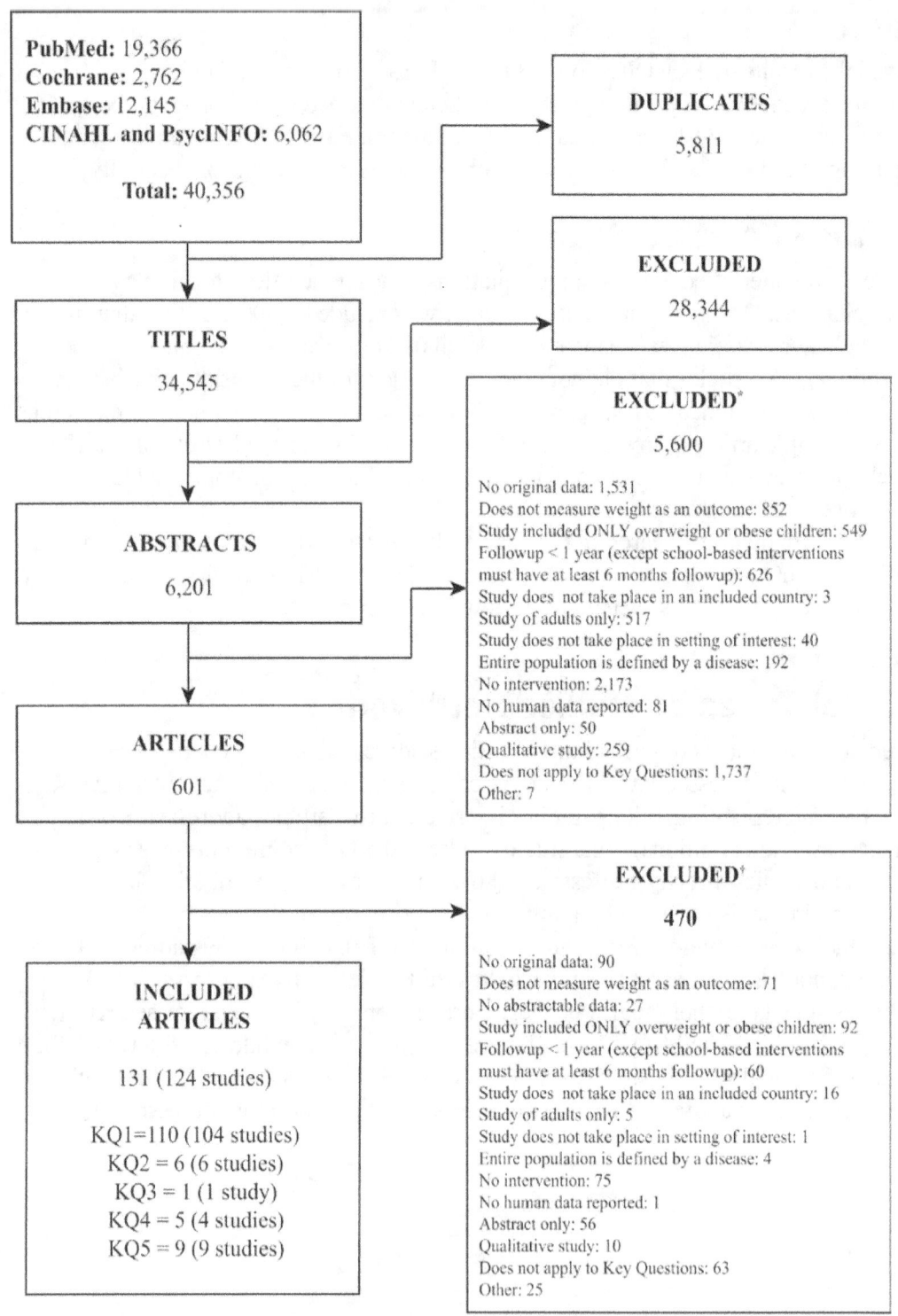

PubMed: 19,366
Cochrane: 2,762
Embase: 12,145
CINAHL and PsycINFO: 6,062

Total: 40,356

DUPLICATES
5,811

EXCLUDED
28,344

TITLES
34,545

EXCLUDED*
5,600

No original data: 1,531
Does not measure weight as an outcome: 852
Study included ONLY overweight or obese children: 549
Followup < 1 year (except school-based interventions must have at least 6 months followup): 626
Study does not take place in an included country: 3
Study of adults only: 517
Study does not take place in setting of interest: 40
Entire population is defined by a disease: 192
No intervention: 2,173
No human data reported: 81
Abstract only: 50
Qualitative study: 259
Does not apply to Key Questions: 1,737
Other: 7

ABSTRACTS
6,201

ARTICLES
601

EXCLUDED†
470

No original data: 90
Does not measure weight as an outcome: 71
No abstractable data: 27
Study included ONLY overweight or obese children: 92
Followup < 1 year (except school-based interventions must have at least 6 months followup): 60
Study does not take place in an included country: 16
Study of adults only: 5
Study does not take place in setting of interest: 1
Entire population is defined by a disease: 4
No intervention: 75
No human data reported: 1
Abstract only: 56
Qualitative study: 10
Does not apply to Key Questions: 63
Other: 25

INCLUDED ARTICLES

131 (124 studies)

KQ1=110 (104 studies)
KQ2 = 6 (6 studies)
KQ3 = 1 (1 study)
KQ4 = 5 (4 studies)
KQ5 = 9 (9 studies)

*Sum of excluded abstracts exceeds 5,600 because reviewers were not required to agree on reasons for exclusion.
†Sum of excluded abstracts exceeds 470 because reviewers were not required to agree on reasons for exclusion.

KQ 1: What is the comparative effectiveness of school-based interventions for the prevention of obesity or overweight in children?

Key Points

School-Only–Based Studies

The strength of evidence is moderate that diet or physical activity interventions are more effective at preventing obesity and insufficient that a combination of diet and physical activity is more effective at preventing obesity or overweight than the control.

Heterogeneity of outcomes graded to determine strength of evidence in combination diet and physical activity settings prevented us from conducting a true meta-analysis for this intervention. We analyzed studies with sufficient data to determine impact on BMI and BMI z-score and found that these specific outcomes were positively impacted.

School-Home–Based Studies

Only one study investigated the effectiveness of a diet intervention on obesity prevention. This RCT, with 1,321 students, demonstrated a significant decrease in the prevalence of overweight and obese children as a result of the intervention. However, since there is only one study, and the risk of bias is moderate, the strength of the evidence is insufficient that diet interventions are more effective in preventing obesity or overweight than the control.

Of the three physical activity intervention studies that measured change in BMI, all showed a statistically significant reduction in the intervention group relative to the control group. The strength of the evidence is high that physical activity interventions are more effective in preventing obesity or overweight than the control intervention.

Twenty-seven studies conducted in both the school and home settings implemented interventions of both diet and physical activity. Among these 27 studies, 21 demonstrated a favorable effect of the intervention on weight outcomes compared to the control. However, only 10 of the studies had statistically significant results. The strength of the evidence is moderate that diet and physical activity-combined interventions are more effective in preventing obesity and overweight than the control.

School-Home-Community–Based Studies

Out of nine studies, two studies in this setting showed a significant desirable effect on obesity prevention, both of which intervened on a combination of diet and physical activity.

The strength of evidence is insufficient that physical activity interventions are more effective at preventing obesity or overweight than the control, based on one non-RCT study.

The strength of evidence is high that combined diet and physical activity interventions are more effective at preventing obesity or overweight than the control, based on four RCTs and four non-RCTs. Among those reported, around half found desirable and significant changes in BMI, BMI z-score, prevalence of overweight or obesity, percentage of body fat, and waist circumference.

School-Community–Based Studies

Out of six studies in this setting, two showed a significant desirable effect: one intervened on diet, and the other intervened on a combination of diet and physical activity.

The strength of evidence is insufficient that a diet intervention is more effective at preventing obesity or overweight than the control, based on one RCT. The single study did show significant lower incidence rate for overweight in the intervention as compared to the control (p=0.018).

The strength of the evidence is moderate that combined diet and physical activity interventions is more effective at preventing obesity or overweight than the control, based on one RCT and three non-RCTs. The two studies with moderate risk of bias showed a favorable effect and there was no other low risk of bias studies in the opposite direction.

The strength of the evidence is insufficient that a physical activity and self-management intervention is more effective at preventing obesity or overweight than the control, based on one RCT. This study shows no difference between the intervention and control groups.

School-Consumer Health Informatics–Based Studies

Four studies took place in this setting. The evidence is insufficient that school with consumer health informatics physical activity or combined diet and physical activity interventions prevent obesity or overweight in children.

School-Home-Consumer Health Informatics–Based Studies

One study took place in this setting. The evidence is insufficient that school, home, consumer health informatics combination diet and physical activity interventions prevent obesity or overweight in children.

School-Only–Based Studies

Study Characteristics

Fifty-four studies, described in 58 articles reported on school-only-based interventions. Thirty-six of these studies were RCTs. Twenty-three of the RCTs had a stated goal of obesity prevention in children.[45-63] Thirteen RCTs took place in the U.S.[45,46,48,50,56,57,64-70] The remaining RCTs took place in Australia, Belgium, Canada, the Northern Marianas, France, Germany, Greece, Iceland, Italy, New Zealand, Poland, Portugal, Spain, Switzerland, and the United Kingdom (Table 3; Appendix E, Evidence Table 1).

Seven RCTs (19.4 percent) did not specify inclusion or exclusion criteria.[51,56,65,71-74] Three RCT's included girls only,[50,60,68] two RCT's included boys only,[57,59] and the remainder did not use sex as an exclusion criteria. Of the eight RCTs that used age range as an inclusion criteria, one included only children under 5 years old,[75] two included children ages 5 to 7 years,[53,58] two included children ages 6 to 10 years,[63,76] one included children ages 7 to 11 years,[49,54] and two included children ages 8 to 12 years.[57,68] Many RCTs used grade level as an inclusion criteria; one included "pre-school" children,[77] eight included children in grades 1, 2, or 3;[45,48,53,58,64,76,78,79] two included children in grades 3 to 5;[57 68] ten included children in grades 4, 5, or 6;[46,52,66,67,69,70,80-83] one included "primary school" children;[47] two included children in grades 7, 8, or 9;[59,60] and one included "junior high school" children.[54] We list additional inclusion criteria in Table 3 and Appendix E, Evidence Table 1.

Eighteen of the school-based studies were non-RCTs: 16 were clinical trials (non-randomized), one was pre-post design, one was a natural experiment, one was a pilot study and two were quasi-experimental. Ten of the non-RCTs had a stated goal of weight maintenance or obesity prevention in children.[84-94] Seven took place in the U.S.,[74,85,86,89,95-97] and the remainder took place in Canada, Germany, Chile, Croatia, Greece, Italy, New Zealand, Norway, Spain and Sweden (Table 3; Appendix E, Evidence Table 1).

Seven of these non-RCTs (39 percent) did not specify inclusion criteria.[85,94,95,97-100] Three included girls only,[92,93,101] and the remainder did not specify any sex for enrollment. Two studies restricted study participation by age, enrolling 9 to 11 year olds,[89] and 16 to 18 year olds.[93] The remainder of the non-RCTs did not limit participation by age. Eleven non-RCTs restricted participation by grade. One limited participation to preschoolers;[102] one to first-graders;[103,104] two to children in grades 1 or 2;[92,101] four to children in grades 3, 4, or 5;[86,90,93,96] one to children in grades 7 thru 9;[91] and one to children in grades 1 to 8.[84] The remaining studies did not limit participation by grade level. Other inclusion criteria are in Table 3 and Appendix E, Evidence Table 1.

Population Characteristics

The number of participants across all RCTs was 31,126; each individual RCT included between 100 and 6,413 participants. Three RCTs included only girls.[50,60,68] The remainder of the RCTs had between 36 and 60 percent girls enrolled or did not report on this characteristic. Seventeen RCTs had participants in elementary grades (ages 6.1 to 9.7 years) (Table 3; Appendix E, Evidence Table 2).[47-49,51,53,55,57,58,61,62,64,66,68,69,73,76,77,79] Thirteen RCTs had participants in middle-school (ages 10 to 15.8 years),[46,50,52,56,59,60,67,70-72,81,83,105] and eight did not report on the age of their participants.[45,54,63,65,74,78,80,82]

There were 18 non-RCTs that included from 77 to 4,500 participants, with 12,405 participants across studies. Of the non-RCTs reporting on sex, three enrolled only girls,[92,93,101] and the others had between 38 and 59.7 percent girls enrolled. Of the non-RCTs reporting on age, all children were between 6 and 15 years old (Table 3; Appendix E, Evidence Table 2).[64,84-87,91,92,95,97-99,101,106]

Fourteen non-RCTs reported on grade range. Twelve included participants in elementary school,[64,85-87,92,94,95,97-99,101,106] four included participants in middle school,[84,88,89,91] and one included participants in grades 2 through 6.[85] The majority of studies did not report on participant race. One non-RCTs had only black non-Hispanic participants,[85] one study had up 94.2 percent Latin/Hispanic participants,[74] three studies had at least 80 percent white non-Hispanic participants,[92,99,106] and one study had a population of mixed races (Table 3; Appendix E, Evidence Table 2).[96]

Interventions

Thirty-six of the 54 studies were RCTs. four RCTs described in four articles had arms that included diet interventions.[49,54,55,64,83] These RCT's were directed at dietary changes and utilized educational interventions.[49,54,55,64,83] Ten RCTs had arms that included physical activity interventions.[45,52,57,73,76,79,80,82,83,105] Of these, one RCT had arms that included education-only interventions,[105] five had arms that included environment-only interventions,[52,57,73,76,79] and four had arms that included both educational and environmental physical activity interventions.[45,80,82,83] Twenty-four RCTs had arms that included both diet and physical activity interventions.[46-48,50,51,53,56,58-63,65-72,74,78,84] Nine RCTs had arms that included a combination of diet, physical activity, and self-management interventions.[46,47,50,55,56,67,70,72,78] One RCT had intervention arms that were dietary interventions only, physical activity interventions only, and a combined diet and physical activity intervention arm.[83] As such, we counted the study in all three categories listed above. Other combinations of interventions are on Table 4 and Appendix E, Evidence Table 3.

No non-RCTs addressed diet interventions. Nine of the 18 non-RCTs tested physical activity interventions.[86,87,92,93,95,96,98,101,106] One arm included educational intervention only,[95] six had arms that included environmental interventions only,[87,92,93,98,101,106] and the remainder included both educational and environmental interventions.[86,96] Ten non-RCTs had arms that included diet and physical activity (Table 4; Appendix E, Evidence Table 3).[74,84,85,88,90,91,94,97,99,100,103,104]

Table 3. Study and participant characteristics of studies based only in schools

Author, Year	RCT	Goal: Obesity Prevention	Country	Sex*	Age Range, Years*	Grade*	Other*	Total N	Followup in Weeks†	% Girls†	Mean Age [Range] Years†	Grade†	Race†
Amaro, 2006[72]	Y	N	Italy	NR	NR	NR	NR	241	26	44.8	11-14	Middle school	WNH 100
Barbeau, 2007[68]	Y	N	U.S.	NR	8-12	3,4,5	BNH, <300 lbs., no meds, regular physical activity	201	43	100	9.5	Elementary school	BNH 100
Bronikowski, 2011[105]	Y	N	Poland	NR	NR	NR	NR	137	130	NR	13.2	NR	NR
Burguera, 2011[91]	N	Y	Spain	NR	NR	7-9	Could not be part of any federated sport team or organized after-school sports.	90	26	59.7	13.9	NR	NR
Bush, 1989[70]	Y	N	U.S.	NR	NR	4-6	NR	1,041	104	54	10.5	NR	NR
Chiodera, 2008[106]	N	N	Italy	NR	NR	NR	BMI<30, no major pathologies, no outside physical activity	4,500	34	50.1	6-10	Primary school	NR
Coleman, 2011[64]	Y	N	U.S.	NR	NR	2, 3, 6	NR	NR	104	57	8.9	NR	Mixed
Damon, 2005[94]	N	Y	Austria	NR	NR	NR	NR	481	43	NR	10-12	1	NR

Table 3. Study and participant characteristics of studies based only in schools (continued)

Author, Year	RCT	Goal: Obesity Prevention	Country	Sex*	Age Range, Years*	Grade*	Other*	Total N	Followup in Weeks†	% Girls†	Mean Age [Range] Years†	Grade†	Race†
DeBar, 2011[65]	Y	N	U.S.	NR	NR	6	Schools were at least 50% of students were eligible for welfare, black, or Hispanic.	4603	104	Arm1: 46.5 Arm2: 58.6 Arm3: 49.3	11.2-11.3	NR	Mixed
Donnelly, 2009[45]	Y	Y	U.S.	NR	NR	2&3	NR	1,527	156	51.7	NR	NR	Mixed (all)
Foster, 2012[46]	Y	Y	U.S.	NR	NR	6	50% of children in the school needed to be eligible for federally subsidized lunches; 50% of the students had to be black or Hispanic	4,603	156	52.7	11.3	6	Hispanic: 54.2 Black: 18.0 White: 19.3 Other: 8.5
Fung, 2012[90]	N	Y	Canada	NR	NR	5	NR	NR	104		NR	5	NR
Gortmaker, 1999[56]	Y	Y	U.S.	NR	NR	NR	NR	1,295	104	Arm1: 50.7 Arm2: 48.5	11.7	NR	Mixed (all)
Graf, 2008[47]	Y	Y	Germany	NR	NR	Primary school	NR	615	208	48.9	6.8	Primary school	NR
Gutin, 2008[48]	Y	Y	U.S.	NR	NR	3	NR	210	138	53	8.5	3	BNH >50
Haerens, 2006[71]	Y	N	Belgium	NR	NR	NR	NR	2,840	95	36.6	13.06	7-8	NR
Heelan, 2009[95]	Y	N	U.S.	NR	NR	NR	NR	324	78	55	8.3	1-5	NR
Howe, 2011[57]	Y	Y	U.S.	Boys	8-12	3-5	Weigh <300lbs Not taking medication No physical impairment to regular PA	106	40	NR	9.7-9.9	3-5	BNH 100
Jago, 2011[81]	Y	N	U.S.	NR	NR	6	NR	6,413	NR	52.4	11.3	NR	Mixed (all)

22

Table 3. Study and participant characteristics of studies based only in schools (continued)

Author, Year	RCT	Goal: Obesity Prevention	Country	Sex*	Age Range, Years*	Grade*	Other*	Total N	Followup in Weeks†	% Girls†	Mean Age [Range] Years†	Grade†	Race†
James, 2004[49]	Y	Y	U.K.	NR	7-11	NR	Parental consent	644	52	50	8.7	NR	NR
James, 2007[54]	Y	Y	U.K.	NR	7-11	Jr. high school	NR	644	39	50	NR	NR	NR
Kafatos, 2005[78]	Y	N	Greece	NR	NR	1	NR	541	312	NR	NR	NR	NR
Kain, 2009[84]	N	Y	Chile	NR	NR	1-8	NR	2,430	314	38	10	NR	NR
Klish, 2012[74]	N	N	U.S.	NR	NR	3-5	NR	1,289	36	Arm1: 49.4 Arm2: 46.3	7.86-7.95	NR	Latin/ Hispanic >92
Lazaar, 2007[79]	Y	N	France	NR	NR	1,2	No know disease, no other studies	425	26	50	7.4	NR	NR
Llargues, 2012[58]	Y	Y	Spain	NR	5-6	1	No special diet, no physical activity incapacities	509	208	Arm1: 45.6 Arm2: 46.3	6-8	NR	NR
Lubans, 2012[59]	Y	Y	Australia	Boys	NR	9	Speak English	100	24	NR	14.3	9	NR
Lubans, 2012[60]	Y	Y	Australia	Girls	NR	8	Low SES	357	52	100	13.8	8	Australian 85.4 Asian 1.1 European 10.1
Madsen, 1993[67]	Y	N	U.S.	NR	NR	5, 6	No high BP, no CVD, no high cholesterol	314	104	NR	12	5-6	NR
Magnusson, 2012[61]	Y	Y	Iceland	NR	NR	NR	Born in 1999	266	NR	Arm1: 60 Arm2: 51	7.3-7.4	NR	WNH 100
Manios, 1999[103]	N	N	Greece	NR	NR	1	NR	1,046	156	NR	NR	NR	NR
Manios, 2002[104]	N	N	Greece	NR	NR	1	NR	1,046	312	47	NR	NR	NR
Manios, 2006[100]	N	N	Greece	NR	NR	NR	NR	441	312	NR	NR	1-5	NR
Metcalf, 2012[77]	Y	Y	Switzerland	NR	NR	Pre-school	NR	652	47	50	5.2	NR	NR

23

Table 3. Study and participant characteristics of studies based only in schools (continued)

Author, Year	RCT	Goal: Obesity Prevention	Country	Sex*	Age Range, Years*	Grade*	Other*	Total N	Followup in Weeks†	% Girls†	Mean Age [Range] Years†	Grade†	Race†
Muckelbauer, 2009[55]	Y	Y	Germany	NR	NR	NR	School level randomization	3,190	NR	49.7	8.3	2-3	NR
Neumark-Sztainer, 2010[50]	Y	Y	U.S.	Girls	NR	NR	No high-level physical activity, no eating disorder	356	36-52	100	15.8	NR	Mixed (all)
Newton, 2010[85]	N	Y	U.S.	NR	NR	NR	NR	77	78	50	9.26	2-6	BNH 100
Reed, 2008[82]	Y	N	Canada	NR	NR	4- 5	No health condition limiting physical activity	268	NR	NR	NR	NR	NR
Resaland, 2011[87]	N	N	Norway	NR	NR	4	NR	256	104	Arm1: 57 Arm2: 56	9.2	NR	NR
Rosario, 2012[82]	Y	Y	Portugal	NR	NR	NR	Attend public elementary schools	464	24	51.5	8.3	NR	NR
Rush, E, 2012[63]	Y	Y	New Zealand	NR	5-10	NR	NR	NR	104	50.2	NR	NR	European 67.3; Maori 25.7; Others 7
Sahota, 2001[51]	Y	Y	U.K.	NR	NR	NR	NR	636	NR	NR	8.3	4-5	NR
Sallis, 1993[86]	Y	Y	U.S.	NR	NR	4	NR	549	NR	44	9.25	4	WNH >80
Sallis, 2003[75]	Y	N	US	NR	>5	NR	NR	1,858	156	48.2	7.7	NR	Mixed (All)
Salmon, 2008[80]	Y	Y	Australia	NR	NR	5	Low SES	306	39	51	NR	NR	NR
Scheffler 2007[102]	N	N	Germany	NR	NR	Pre-school	NR	264	104	NR	NR	NR	NR
Skybo, 2002[96]	N	N	U.S.	NR	NR	NR	English speakers	58	39	48	NR	3	Mixed (all)
Smolak, 2001[89]	N	N	U.S.	NR	9-11	NR	NR	509	104	49.5	NR	6	NR
Sollerhed, 2008[98]	Y	Y	Sweden	NR	NR	NR	NR	132	156	44.6	6-9	NR	NR

Table 3. Study and participant characteristics of studies based only in schools (continued)

Author, Year	RCT	Goal: Obesity Prevention	Country	Sex*	Age Range, Years*	Grade*	Other*	Total N	Followup in Weeks†	% Girls†	Mean Age [Range] Years†	Grade†	Race†
Stenevi-Lundgren, 2009[92]	N	N	Sweden	Girls	NR	1-2	Healthy girls, no meds	103	52-104 (Control group was followed for 104)	100	7.9	1-2	WNH 100
Stock, 2007[88]	N	Y	Canada	NR	NR	NR	School-level randomization	360	43	55.2	NR	7-8	NR
Taylor, 2007[99]	N	Y	New Zealand	NR	NR	NR	NR	730	104	49.8	7.7	NR	WNH >80
Thivel, 2011[76]	Y	N	France	NR	6-10	1 or 2	No more than 3 hours physical activity per day, no known disease, no other studies	457	26	52	6-10	1-2	NR
Treveno, 2005[69]	Y	N	U.S.	NR	NR	4	Low income	387	34	52	9.7	NR	NR
Tucker, 2011[97]	N	N	U.S.	NR	NR	NR	NR	99	34	100	9.6	4-5	NR
Valdimarsson, 2006[101]	N	N	Sweden	Girls	NR	1-2	NR	103	52–104†	100	7.8	NR	NR
Vandongen, 1995[83]	Y	N	Australia	NR	NR	8	NR	1,147	39	42.2	10-12	6	NR
Vizcaino, 2008[73]	Y	Y	Spain	NR	NR	NR	NR	1,044	36-72	54	9.4	NR	NR
Walter, 1985[66]	Y	N	U.S.	NR	NR	4	NR	1,563	52	48.6	9.1	4	Mixed (all)
Walther, 2009[52]	Y	N	Germany	NR	NR	6	NR	211	52	45	11.1	6	NR
Warren, 2003[53]	Y	Y	U.S.	NR	5-7	Primary school	NR	218	61-69	49	6.1	1-2	NR

AIAN = American Indian/Alaska Native; API = Asian Pacific Islander; BMI = Body Mass Index (in kg/m^2); BNH = Black Non-Hispanic; BP = Blood Pressure; CVD = Cardio Vascular Disease; Maint = Maintenance; Meds = Medications; N = No; NR = Not Reported; physical activity = Physical Activity; RCT = Randomized Controlled Trials; WNH = White Non-Hispanic; Y=Yes
*Inclusion/exclusion criteria.
†Participant characteristics.

25

Table 4. Interventions of studies based only in schools

Author, Year	Control Arm	Description of Intervention	Diet (Phys/Env)	Diet (Psych)	Physical Activity (Phys/Env)	Physical Activity (Psych)
Amaro, 2006[72]	Usual care	Kaledo: Educational board-game on Mediterranean diet with one play session per week and one PA session per week, also includes BMI screening.		X	X	
Barbeau, 2007[68]	Usual care	Subjects given healthy snacks during homework time, and a PA component including skills development, MVPA, and heart rate monitors.	X		X	
Bronikowski, 2011[105]	Usual care	PE teachers provided social support and reinforcement for student's self-programmed out-of-school physical activity plan. Those pupils who fulfilled the PA obligations in PA plan received a reward.			X	
Burguera, 2011[91]	Despite informed consent, did not participate in the intervention	ACTYBOSS: Subjects offered two nutrition and behavioral modification workshops. Special emphasis on healthy lifestyle and self-responsibility. Opportunities to participate in PA sessions, not stated if required.		X	X	X
Bush, 1989[70]	Parents only received results of screening	Subjects received nutrition, exercise, anti-smoking lessons, health screening and a "Health Passport". Health newsletters were mailed to parents throughout intervention	X	X		
Chiodera, 2008[106]	No control	Aimed to professionally qualify PE in schools without changing hours dedicated per week			X	
Coleman, 2011[64]	Usual care	Healthy ONES: Subjects brought unhealthy snacks from home. Subjects discouraged from unhealthy snacks by teachers and staff, including promoting healthy eating in class. More nutritious snacks and food offered at school, especially for events.	X	X		
Damon, 2005[94]	Usual care	Education on diet and physical activity and increase in physical activity	X		X	X
DeBar, 2011[65]	Usual care	1 hour initial training outlined the required tasks, skills, and procedures, including 30-minute trainings specific to each intervention activity. Communications intervention strategies, including public commitment opportunities for students, were intended to strengthen the impact of all HEALTHY intervention components. Themes included healthier diet, decrease sugar drinks and increase PA.		X	X	X
Donnelly, 2009[45]	Usual care	A target goal of 90min/week of MVPA per child was given along with WSB to increase frequency of walking to school. Teacher training was implemented for the intervention			X	X

26

Table 4. Interventions of studies based only in schools (continued)

Author, Year	Control Arm	Description of Intervention	Diet (Phys/Env)	Diet (Psych)	Physical Activity (Phys/Env)	Physical Activity (Psych)
Foster, 2010[46]	Usual care	Quantity and nutritional quality of food served in the school environment was changed. The amount of time students spent in moderate to vigorous physical activity was increased. Behavioral knowledge and skill were taught in classrooms using the FLASH program	X		X	
Fung, 2012[90]	Usual care	APPLE: School health facilitators promote community gardens and healthier breakfast/lunch options. Facilitated professional development for teachers and school staff, and parent information nights. After school PA sessions promoted along with walk to school days. Weekend events, celebrations and newsletters used to promote healthy living.	X		X	
Gortmaker, 1999[56]	Usual care	Planet Health: Class sessions focused on behavioral changes to promote healthy eating, MVPA, and reduce TV time.		X	X	
Graf, 2008[47]	Usual care	Extra health education on nutrition, biology, self-management. PA breaks were provided in mornings.		X	X	X
Gutin, 2008[48]	Regular health screening and diet/PA information included	Youths were provided healthy snacks during after-school PA sessions along with academic enrichment homework and assistance.	X		X	
Haerens, 2006[71]	Usual care	Subjects received additional information on healthy living along with providing healthy snack options. For PA, a computer tailored intervention was implemented about the child's activity levels and feedback. Schools were encouraged to offer more PA opportunities. Newsletters were sent out to community and parents regarding the intervention.	X	X	X	X
Heelan, 2009[95]	Usual care	Walking School Bus program. Children walk in groups along set route to school, with adult as "driver" (chaperone).			X	
Howe, 2011[57]	Usual care	After school program for two hours that included; skills development, VPA, toning and stretching			X	
James, 2004[49] James, 2007[54]	Usual care	Discourage drinking of fizzy drinks (sweetened and unsweetened) among school-age children.		X		

Table 4. Interventions of studies based only in schools (continued)

Author, Year	Control Arm	Description of Intervention	Diet (Phys/Env)	Diet (Psych)	Physical Activity (Phys/Env)	Physical Activity (Psych)
Kafatos, 2005[78]	Usual care	Cretan Health/Nutrition Program: Classroom modules designed to develop behavioral capability, expectations, and self-efficacy for healthy eating. Theoretical component of PA was given by PE instructor along with PA sessions. Children also kept food diary.		X	X	X
Kain, 2009[84]	Usual care	Intervention included diet/nutrition lessons and additional PE sessions along with novel card game to promote healthy living.		X	X	
Klish, 2012[74]	Usual care	Obese children with parents were invited to after-school behavior modification program that offered dietary instruction and behavioral therapy. Chef-in-school program: professional chef comes to the school to teach how to prepare healthy meals. New exercise equipment brought in to promote active recess time.		X	X	
Lazaar, 2007[79]	Usual care	After school PA program with double objective; playful physical practice and dynamic exercise within 1 hour.			X	
Llargues, 2012[58]	Usual care	IVAC method: Promoting healthy dietary habits and increasing PA through pedagogy Investigation, Vision, Action and Change intervention (IVAC)		X		
Lubans, 2012[59]	Usual care	PALs: Nutritional handbooks and seminars, sport sessions, lunchtime activities and leadership sessions.		X	X	X
Lubans, 2012[60]	Usual care	Nutritional handbooks and seminars, sport sessions, lunchtime activities and leadership sessions.		X	X	X
Madsen, 1993[67]	No control	SCORES: Children in program pay soccer three days a week, community service and/or creative writing. Training in self-monitoring in regard to diet and sodium content along with self-monitoring for PA.		X	X	X
Magnusson, 2012[61]	Usual care	Interventions were designed to increase dietary knowledge and self-efficacy. Teachers integrated PA into curriculum.		X	X	
Manios, 1999[103] Manios, 2002[104] Manios, 2006[100]	Usual care for children, and parents received mailed envelopes with all medical screening results with brief comments	Educational sessions offered for health and nutritional components. PA component included educational sessions and increased PA with stretching, fitness stations and aerobic games.		X	X	X

Table 4. Interventions of studies based only in schools (continued)

Author, Year	Control Arm	Description of Intervention	Diet (Phys/Env)	Diet (Psych)	Physical Activity (Phys/Env)	Physical Activity (Psych)
Muckelbauer, 2009[55]	Usual care	Intervention targeted behavioral change and education regarding diet, nutrition, and goal setting.	X	X		
Neumark-Sztainer, 2010[50]	Usual care	New Moves: intervention targets increasing fruit, vegetable intake, and limiting sugar-sweetened beverages. Subjects were served healthy foods during lunch and offered more PA opportunities	X	X	X	
Newton, 2010[85]	No control	School Cafeteria were modified with more healthy choices up to the state standards. Teachers were encouraged to model daily PA tips for short bouts of PA and an additional increased PE session indoors.	X	X	X	X
Reed, 2008[82]	Usual care	Goal to deliver 15 min of MVPA daily for 75 extra min of PA per week in schools. Principals and teachers met with facilitators to design program. Teachers also provide classroom activities such as skipping, dancing and resistance training.			X	X
Resaland, 2011[87]	Usual care	60 min of PA conducted by specialist PE teacher for 104 weeks			X	
Rosario, 2012[62]	Usual care	Teachers addressed nutrition topics via classroom activities, including food, nutrition, diet guidelines, along with PA/lifestyle topics.		X	X	X
Rush, 2012[63]	Usual care	Energizer educated through information regarding replacing sugary drinks with water and importance of eating breakfast. Canteen makeovers were conducted to remove pastries and pies, and to add healthier options. Promotion of PA sessions with games and activities.	X	X	X	X
Sahota, 2001[51]	Usual care	Increase knowledge and attitudes towards healthy living, modification of school meals and PE sessions.	X	X	X	
Sallis, 1993[86]	Usual care	Self-management program to promote PA outside school for children. Lessons taught skills to maintain activity habits post-intervention. Additional PE classes were provided. A brief nutrition intervention of seminars for teachers were also conducted			X	X
Salmon, 2008[80]	Usual care	BM/FMS: Focused on teaching object control and locomotors skills. Reduce TV and video game time at home and involvement of parents in process.			X	X
Skybo, 2002[96]	Usual care	American Heart Association Heart Power! Emphasize nutrition in class discussions as well as importance of PA. Children then engaged in PA such as jumping jacks or running in place.		X	X	X

29

Table 4. Interventions of studies based only in schools (continued)

Author, Year	Control Arm	Description of Intervention	Diet (Phys/Env)	Diet (Psych)	Physical Activity (Phys/Env)	Physical Activity (Psych)
Smolak, 2001[89]	No curriculum different schools	ESEM: Encouraged parents to modify diet and PA habits at home.			X	X
Sollerhed, 2008[98]	Usual care	I-school: Increased PE time in intervention school, time was expanded from one/two lessons per week to 4 lessons			X	
Stenevi-Lundgren, 2009[92]	Usual care	Increase school PE time per week.			X	
Stock, 2007[88]	Usual care	Themes targeted exposure to nutritional information on foods and beverages. Themes also included structured PA/aerobic fitness and lessons on healthy body image and self-esteem.		X	X	X
Taylor, 2007[99]	Usual care	APPLE: Encourage healthy eating with science lessons highlighting adverse health effects of sugary drinks and fatty foods. Cooled water filters installed in schools to promote drinking water. Initiatives were set to promote more PA activity as well as sports equipment were provided for free time.	X	X	X	X
Thivel, 2011[76]	Usual care	PA program of additional 2hrs of PA in addition to 2hrs of regular PE class. Objective to increase PA and minimize inactivity			X	
Trevino, 2005[69]	Usual care	Beinestar Health Program: Decrease dietary fats and increase fiber intake through parent fun activities. PA promotion was also included in the activities along with a after school program with activities such as games, dancing, singing, crafts, etc.		X	X	X
Tucker, 2011[97]	Let's Go 5-2-1-0 Program curriculum ONLY, without student nurse coaching, parent evening offerings, and reinforcement incentives	Let's Go: Coaching sessions designed to promote healthy eating and exercise conducted by nursing staff and parents.		X		X
Valdimarsson, 2006[101]	Usual care	POP: Increase PA in schools from 60min/week to 200min/week.			X	
Vandongen, 1995[83]	Usual care	Increase fruit and vegetable consumption and whole grains while also reducing consumption of fatty foods and sugar sweetened beverages with educational lessons		X		
Vandongen, 1995[83]	Usual care	Classroom sessions providing rational basis for activity programs. Fitness program included relays, skipping and health hustles.			X	X

30

Table 4. Interventions of studies based only in schools (continued)

Author, Year	Control Arm	Description of Intervention	Diet (Phys/Env)	Diet (Psych)	Physical Activity (Phys/Env)	Physical Activity (Psych)
Vandongen, 1995[83]	Usual care	Classroom sessions to provide rational basis for activity programs. Activity programs include; relays, skipping and health hustles. Heart rates of 150-170 beats/min were to be achieved in first 15 min. Nutrition education was provided focusing on increase fruits, vegetables, whole grains, and decrease intake of fatty foods and sugars. Homework assignments and comics were given to children to help improve healthy eating.		X	X	X
Vizcaino, 2008[73]	Usual care	Activity program with sports using alternative equipment (pogo sticks, Frisbees, parachutes, etc.). Primary care providers encouraged to focus on behavioral targets for patients			X	
Walter, 1985[66]	Usual care	Incorporates social learning strategies to encourage behavioral change regarding diet and PA (improvement of cardiovascular fitness)		X		X
Walther, 2009[52]	Mandatory 2 units (45 mins.) of PE classes/week plus healthy lifestyle lessons/month	45 min of PA with 15 min endurance training per school day. Non-randomized sport students received 12 units (45min) of high-level endurance exercise per week.			X	
Warren, 2003[53]	Be smart; educational program about food in non-nutrition sense.	Eat Smart Educational Intervention: emphasizing food contributing to health and healthy food. Lessons were given in PA education and television viewing.		X		X

Phys/Env=Physical/environmental intervention; Psych = psychosocial intervention

31

Outcomes

Diet Interventions
We identified two RCTs, described in three articles.[49,54,83]

Weight-Related Outcomes

BMI z-Score
One study reported on BMI z-score showing a significant decrease of it at final followup at 158 weeks (mean difference=0.24; 95% CI: 0.02 to .46; p=0.03)[49,54] (Appendix E, Evidence Table 4a).

BMI
Both of the diet intervention studies reported on BMI as an outcome. One study looked at the entire population and showed significant changes in BMI in favor of the intervention group at 158 weeks (mean difference =0.68; 95% CI: 0.06 to 1.30; p=0.03).[49,54] One study reported on a subgroup analyses by sex. The results showed a nonsignificant change in favor of the control for boys, and nonsignificant change in favor of the intervention for girls (Appendix E, Evidence Table 4a,b).[83]

Prevalence of Overweight and Obesity
One study reported on prevalence of obesity and overweight, but found no statistical significance intervention effect.[49,54] The study reported prevalence of overweight and obesity in subgroups of boys and girls and found no intervention effect (Appendix E, Evidence Table 4a,b).[49,54]

Percent Body Fat
One study reported percent body fat change in subgroups of boys and girls. In both subgroups the there was no intervention effect (Appendix E, Evidence Table 4b).[83]

Waist Circumference
One study reported on waist circumference.[54] This study showed a change in waist circumference in favor of the intervention, but it was not significant (Appendix E, Evidence Table 4a).

Skinfold Thickness
One study reported on skinfold thickness in subgroups by sex. The changes in triceps skinfold thickness in boys favored the control and for girls, favored the intervention. Neither difference was significant.[83] The change in subscapular skinfold thickness favored the control for both the boys and girls. Neither difference was significant (Appendix E, Evidence Table 4b).[83]

Clinical Outcomes
One study reported on systolic and diastolic blood pressure in boys and girls subgroups. Both controls and interventions decreased for these two outcomes, the differences between the interventions and controls was not significant except in the case of diastolic blood pressure in girls where the difference in decrease was significantly in favor of the intervention (numbers not reported).[83] This study also reported on total cholesterol in boys and girls and found that total

cholesterol was significantly higher in the intervention groups of both the boys and the girls (numbers not reported) (Appendix E, Evidence Table 4c).[83]

Adverse Events
The research did not report any.

Intermediate Outcomes

Dietary Intake
One study examined the change in energy intake using a number of parameters.[83] The percent of energy from sugar decreased significantly in boys, but did not in girls. The percent of energy from total fat increased in the intervention groups relative to the control groups, but was not significant for either boys or girls. For percent of energy intake as saturated fat, the intervention had no effect on boys, but there was a nonsignificant decrease in the intervention girls. Overall energy intake (MJ/d) did not differ between the intervention and control groups for both the boys and girls (Appendix E, Evidence Table 4d).

One study recorded change in carbonated beverage consumption but the differences between groups were not significant (Appendix E, Evidence Table 4d).[49]

Interpretation
The results from an outcome measure from each of the two studies reporting on dietary interventions support our conclusions. One reported on BMI z-score.[54] This study showed a significant decrease in BMI z-score at 3 years. The other study reported on BMI, and showed a nonsignificant change in favor of the intervention in boy and girl subgroups at nine months.[83] Based on this evidence we conclude that dietary interventions positively impact BMI z-score and BMI outcomes. One of these dietary intervention studies has a goal of obesity prevention.[49,54] Both studies focused on education that promoted a healthy diet, and reduced the consumption of carbonated drinks.

Physical Activity Interventions
Fifteen studies reported on the effects of physical activity interventions on weight-related outcomes.[45,52,73,76,79,80,82,83,86,87,89,92,95,101,106]

Weight-Related Outcomes

BMI z-Score
Two studies reported on BMI z-score and found a difference in BMI in the intervention group compared with control groups.[79,95] One study reported a reduction in BMI z-score in favor of the intervention that was not significant.[95] The other study reported reductions in BMI z-score in both boys and girls stratified by obese and non-obese, but these reductions were not significant (Appendix E, Evidence Table 5a,b).[79].

BMI
Six studies reported on BMI in the whole population.[45,52,82,87,92,95] None of these studies found a statistically significant intervention effect. One study showed a nonsignificant reduction in BMI in favor of the intervention group,[52] and two studies showed no difference in BMI between the control and intervention (Appendix E, Evidence Table 5a,b).[45,87]

Nine studies reported on BMI by subgroup. Seven of these studies reported boy and girl subgroups. Six studies reported nonsignificant BMI change in favor of the intervention in boys,[79,83,86,87,89,106] and five studies reported nonsignificant BMI change in favor of the intervention in girls.[79,83,87,106,107] One study reported on BMI change in favor of the control group in boys,[108] and another study reported the same in girls.[86] One study reported a null affect in girls.[108] Another study showed significant changes in BMI in favor of the intervention girls (-0.15; 95%CI: -0.31 to -0.0; p<0.05).[80]

One study reported BMI outcomes by obese and normal weight subgroups, the change was in favor of the intervention, but was not significant in both groups.[76] One study reported on BMI by grade and reported a nonsignificant BMI change in favor of the intervention in most grades (Appendix E, Evidence Table 5a,b).[106]

BMI Percentile

One study reported on BMI percentiles.[95] This study showed a nonsignificant reduction in BMI percentile in favor of the intervention. (Appendix E, Evidence Table 5a).

Prevalence of Overweight and Obesity

Two studies reported on the prevalence of overweight. One study showed a large decrease in obesity prevalence over time, but the significance was not reported in the paper.[52] One study reported on a subgroups of boys and girls, stratified into obese and non-obese groups, with a nonsignificant reduction in the prevalence of overweight among girls and boys in favor of the intervention (Appendix E, Evidence Table 5a,b).[79]

Percent Body Fat

Three studies reported on percent body fat as an outcome in the whole population.[95,101,106] One study showed an increase in body fat in both the intervention and control, but the change was in favor of the control group and was not significant.[92] A second study suggested that the change in percent body fat favors the intervention group, but was not significant.[95] The third study included reported a significant increase in body fat in the intervention group (mean difference =0.9+/- 1.5; p> 0.001).[101] One study reported on percent body fat in boy and girl subgroups. Both subgroups reported changes in favor of the intervention, but they were not significant (Appendix E, Evidence Table 5a,b).[73,83]

Waist Circumference

Two studies reported on waist circumference. One study evaluated the entire population and found a smaller increase in the intervention groups when compared to the control groups.[87] These differences were not significant. A third study evaluated the effect of physical activity on subgroups of boys and girls.[79] This study reported a decrease in two of the intervention groups in boys, but the differences were not significantly different than those seen in the control group. This study did show a significant decrease in waist circumference in the subgroup of obese girls in favor of the intervention (mean difference in difference=0.43 cm; p<0.001). (Appendix E, Evidence Table 5a).[79]

Skinfold Thickness

Two studies measured triceps skinfold thickness. One found a significant difference in triceps skinfold thickness in a subgroup analyses by BMI between the 25th and 75th percentile in favor of the intervention group, (mean difference in differences=-1.25; 95% CI: -1.82 to -0.67; p<0.001) at 52 weeks, but no significant change at 104 weeks.[73] Another found a change in favor of the control for boys and a change in favor of the intervention for girls. Neither of these differences was significant.[83]This same study also reported on subscapular skinfold thickness in the two subgroups and found changes in favor of the intervention, The changes were not significant for either subgroup (Appendix E, Evidence Table 5a,b).[83]

Weight

Three studies reported on weight change. Two studies reported on the entire population and both measured an increase in weight in favor of the control group; increases were not significant in either study.[87,92] Two studies reported on boy and girl subgroups. One study reported no significant change in weight in girls after 104 weeks, however the girls in the intervention group did gain more at the final time point.[108] In the other study reporting on boy and girl subgroups, boys in the intervention group gained less weight at 104 weeks, and girls in the intervention group gained more.[87] The differences were not significant in either subgroup. One study reported on overweight and normal weight subgroups.[76] The normal weight intervention group gained less weight at 26 weeks, and the overweight intervention group gained slightly more at 26 weeks; these changes were not significant (Appendix E, Evidence Table 5a,b).

Clinical Outcomes

Three studies reported on clinical outcomes in the whole population. Two studies reported on systolic and diastolic blood pressure.[82,87]. One study found a significant difference in the systolic blood pressures of children in the intervention group compared with control group (p<0.05 at 39 weeks) but only an nonsignificant decrease in diastolic blood pressure.[82] The other study reported decreases in both systolic and diastolic blood pressure in favor of the intervention that were nonsignificant.[87] One study reported on High-density lipoprotein (HDL) and Low-density lipoprotein (LDL) and reported decreases in both in favor of the intervention that were nonsignificant.[52] Another study reported on LDL, and reported a decrease in favor of the intervention that was not significant.[82] This study also reported on the ration of HLD to LDL and reported a decrease in favor of the intervention that was not significant. Three studies reported total cholesterol. Two studies reported a decrease in favor of the intervention,[82,87] and the third reported a slight decrease in favor of the control which was not significant.[52] Two studies reported changes in triglycerides and reported slight decreases in favor of the intervention, but the decreases were not significant.[52,87] One study reported on clinical outcomes in boy and girl subgroups.[83] The study measured systolic and diastolic blood pressure and total cholesterol. For all of these outcomes, the change in the boys favored the control and were not statistically significant. For the blood pressure outcomes in girls, both favored the intervention and the change in diastolic blood pressure was significantly in favor of the intervention (the paper did not report the p value). Differences in total cholesterol in girls favored the control but differences were nonsignificant (Appendix E, Evidence Table 5c).[83]

Adverse Events

The research did not report any.

Intermediate Outcomes

Physical Activity and Sedentary Behavior

Three studies reported on change in physical activity or sedentary activity. One study reported on reduction of sedentary activity (TV viewing time).[80] This study reported significantly less TV viewing in the intervention group when compared to the control (p<0.05). The three studies measured the change in physical activity in a variety of ways. One study measured daily physical activity using an accelerometer and found a significant increase (p>0.05) in the intervention group when compared to the control.[45] Another study measured change in physical activity in hours per week and found that the intervention group spent significantly more time per week (p>0.05) involved in physical activity than did the control group.[92] This same study looked at participation in organized sports and found that the intervention group spent significantly more time engaged in organized sports (p<0.05) than the control group.[92] One study measured the amount of time spent engaged in moderate activity, and amount of time engaged in vigorous activity.[80] Moderate physical activity increased significantly (p<0.01) in boys engaged in behavior modification and in girls (p<0.05) engaged in movement skills training.[80] Vigorous activity increased significantly in both boys and girls in the intervention groups when compared to no intervention.[80] This same study found that the intervention groups spent significantly less time (p<0.05) watching TV than the control group (Appendix E, Evidence Table 5d).

Interpretation

The results from an outcome measure from each of the 15 studies reporting on physical activity interventions support our conclusions. Two studies reported on BMI z-score.[79,95] Both reported changes in BMI z-score in favor of the intervention. One study did not report on significance,[95] and the other reported an nonsignificant change.[79] Eleven studies reported on BMI.[45,52,76,80,82,83,86,87,89,92,106] Eight of these reported a change in BMI in favor of the intervention. One of these were significant,[80] and the remaining had either nonsignificant changes, or did not report on significance.[52,76,82,87,92,109] A single study reported on change in percent body fat and reported a significant change in favor of the control (no intervention).[101] A single study reported on skinfold thickness fat and reported a significant change in favor of the control (no intervention).[73] Based on this evidence we conclude that physical activity interventions positively impact BMI z-score and BMI. Based on this evidence we cannot conclude that physical activity interventions positively impact skinfold thickness and percent body fat.

One study that showed a significant effect on percent body fat[101] enrolled pre-pubertal girls and focused on daily physical educational classes led by school teachers. A major strength of this study[101] is that we could regard the intervention group as a population-based cohort, since the study invited all girls in grades 1 and 2 in one school enrolled 90 percent.

One study reported on the influence of gender on the magnitude of the changes in anthropometric variables[79] and found a significant reduction in waist circumference of girls but no effect in boys. Plausible explanations for this sex-difference may be that girls are basically less physically active compared to boys; adding daily physical activity into girls' daily routine might have produced a substantial effect on their energy expenditure. Additionally, the post-exercise eating behavior may have been different according to gender.

Some of the physical activity interventions also had impact on clinical outcomes (e.g., systolic blood pressure),[82] and intermediate outcomes (e.g., increasing physical activity and reducing sedentary activities). These studies targeted cardiovascular disease risk profiles[82] and

36

promoted daily physical activity in elementary-school children[45,80,92]. All of these factors may have contributed to the significant effects of the interventions on weight and other outcomes.

There were no clear differences between the studies that were effective at preventing obesity and those that were not.

Diet and Physical Activity Intervention

Thirty-seven studies in 39 articles assessed the effect of a combined diet and physical activity intervention on weight-related outcomes.[47,48,50,51,53,55-72,74,78,83-85,88,90,91,94,96-98,100,103-105]

Weight-Related Outcomes

BMI z-Score

Eleven studies reported on BMI z-score. Seven of these studies reported on BMI z-score in the entire population. Five of these studies reported no significant difference between the intervention and control. Four of these reported increases in BMI z-score in both the intervention and the control but the change favored the intervention.[55,62,72,99] A single study reported no statistics but stated that the difference between the control and intervention was not significant.[51] Another was a pre-post study that reported no statistical change between groups.[85] Two combined diet and physical activity intervention studies that evaluated BMI z-score as an outcome reported a statistically significant change in BMI z-score in favor of the intervention group compared to the control group: mean difference in differences 0.04, p=0.04[46];.mean difference in differences -0.08 (95% CI: -0.02 to 0.04).[60] Four studies that reported on entire populations and BMI z-score were RCTs and included sufficient data and homogeneity for a meta-analysis.[46,55,60,62,72] This analysis showed an overall difference in BMI z-score of -0.08 (95% CI -0.14, -0.02, p=0.009), in favor of the intervention (Figure 3; Appendix E. Evidence Table 6a).

Two studies reporting on BMI z-score also reported data by sex subgroups.[71,84] Both studies reported changes in BMI z-score in favor of the intervention. In one study the changes were significant in favor of the intervention for both subgroups; p<0.05 for both girls and boys[84] The other study found only significant changes in favor of the intervention in girls, p<0.05.[71] (Appendix E. Evidence Table 6b).

BMI

Twenty-one studies, described in 22 articles, reported on BMI. Sixteen of them reported on BMI in the entire population. Seven studies reported no significant intervention effect.[50,57,65,67,91,94,99] Four showed change in BMI in the direction in favor of the intervention,[57,61,65,67,91,99] and one showed no effect in overweight children only.[94] Eight of these studies, described in 11 articles, reported a statistically significant desirable effect on BMI; reported in article with no statistics[48]; adjusted change =-0.45 (95% CI: -0.79 to -0.12); p=0.008;[68]; mean difference in difference at 10 years =0.62; p=0.014[100,103,104]; mean difference in differences =-2; p=0[98]; 0.7 kg/m2 (s.e. 0.28) difference in differences between groups at 4 years; p=0.019[78]; adjusted difference in change = -0.019 (95% CI: -0.70 to 0.33)[60]; mean difference in difference = 0.8; p<0.001[58] However, One study reported a statistically significant change in BMI in favor of the control mean adjusted difference =0.7; p<0.001.[47]

Seven of the studies showing a statistically significant effect were RCTs and included sufficient data for further analysis.[50,57,58,60,61,68,110] These studies showed an overall mean difference of -0.32 kg/m^2 (95% CI: -0.49, -0.16, p<0.001) in favor of intervention (Figure 4; Appendix E. Evidence Table 6a).

Nine studies reporting on BMI also reported data by subgroups. Six by sex,[69,71,78,83,84,105] two by weight status,[47,94] and one by grade.[88] In six of the seven studies, all of the subgroup analyses by sex showed change in BMI in favor of the intervention. One study[105] reported an nonsignificant change in favor of the control, and the other[71] reported an nonsignificant change in BMI in favor of the intervention in girls and a significant change in favor of the intervention in boys (p-value not specified). The studies reporting on weight status subgroups (obese, overweight, underweight, and normal weight) did not report on significance in differences across groups. One found changes in favor of the control in obese, overweight, and normal weight groups, and changes in BMI in favor of the intervention in the underweight group.[47] A study describing grade subgroups reported changes in favor of the intervention, for grades k-3, and a significant difference for grades 4–7; mean difference in differences 0.3, p_0.008 (Appendix E. Evidence Table 6b).[88]

Prevalence of Overweight and Obesity

Eleven studies reported on the prevalence of overweight and obesity. They reported prevalence in one of three ways: prevalence of overweight and obesity, prevalence of obesity, or prevalence of overweight. Four studies reported overweight and obesity prevalence in total populations. Two reported a nonsignificant change in favor of the intervention,[46,58] and another reported a nonsignificant difference in favor of the control.[64] The fourth reported a significant difference in prevalence of overweight/obesity in favor of the intervention; mean difference in differences = 0.31, p=0.04.[55] Five studies reported on the prevalence of obesity in the entire population. All showed a nonsignificant change in obesity prevalence in favor of the intervention.[46,53,62,74,90] Three studies reported on the prevalence of overweight in total populations. One study reported a nonsignificant change in favor of the control,[64] A pre-post study reported no difference,[53] On study, after controlling for confounders, the predicted odds of incidence was 75% lower for the intervention group (odds ratio [OR]: 0.25; 95% CI: 0.07–0.92; p < 0.05) (Appendix E. Evidence Table 6a).[62]

Four studies reported outcomes by sex subgroups. One study reported on prevalence of overweight/obese and found a nonsignificant change in prevalence in favor of the intervention in both boys and girls.[58] Two studies reported on the prevalence of obesity. One study reported a nonsignificant change in prevalence in favor of the intervention for boys, and a significant change in favor of the control for girls; OR, 0.47; 95% CI, 0.24-0.93; p= .03.[56] The other found a significant change in prevalence in favor of the intervention for boys (17.0% to 11.4% vs. 21.6% to 19.7 %, p<0.05) and a nonsignificant change in prevalence in favor of the intervention for girls.[84] One study reported on the prevalence of overweight and showed a nonsignificant change in favor of the intervention for girls and a nonsignificant change in favor of the control for boys (Appendix E, Evidence Table 6b).[78]

Percent Body Fat

Nine studies reported on percentage body fat. They recorded in three ways: percent body fat, percent lean mass, and percent muscle. Six studies reported on percent body fat in the entire population. Three of these studies reported nonsignificant change in body fat in favor of the intervention,[50,61,85] and one showed no significant difference between the intervention and control groups.[96] Two studies reported significant changes in favor of the intervention; adjusted change = _2.01; 95% CI: 2.98 to 1.04; p=0.0001,[68] and p<0.05.[48] One study measured lean mass and reported a nonsignificant change in favor of the control.[61] (Appendix E. Evidence Table 6a).

Four studies presented subgroup results. One study only included girls, and found a nonsignificant change in percent body fat in favor of the intervention.[60] Another reported on percent body fat by age subgroups and found nonsignificant changes in percent body fat in favor of the control group for both 5 to 7 year olds and 10 to 12 year olds.[63] Attendance had a nonsignificant influence on percent body fat in favor of the intervention in one study.[48] One study measured lean muscle mass in boys and girls and there was a significant change in favor of the intervention for boys (p<0.05) and nonsignificant change in favor of the control for girls (Appendix E. Evidence Table 6b).[105]

Waist Circumference

Six studies reported on waist circumference change in the entire population. Five studies reported nonsignificant changes in waist circumference in favor of the intervention.[57,61,68,98,99] One study reported a significant reduction in waist circumference > the 90th percentile (p=0.03) and the same study reported a nonsignificant change in waist circumference in favor of the intervention (Appendix E. Evidence Table 6a).[46]

One study reported on waist circumference based on attendance and found a nonsignificant change in favor of the control.[48] Another study reported on sex subgroups and found significant changes in waist circumference in favor of the intervention group for both boys (p<0.05) and girls (p<0.05) (Appendix E. Evidence Table 6b).[84]

Skinfold Thickness

Studies reported skinfold thickness in two ways: triceps skinfold thickness, and the sum of four skinfold thickness measures. One study reported triceps skinfold thickness for the entire population and showed nonsignificant changes in favor of the intervention.[70] One study reported the sum of four skin fold measures for the entire population and showed a nonsignificant change in favor of the control group (Appendix E. Evidence Table 6a).[61]

Two studies reported on skinfold outcomes in sex subgroups. One study reported on triceps skinfold thickness and showed significant changes in favor of the control in both boys (p<0.05) and girls (p<0.05).[84] Another study reported on the sum of four skinfold measures and found a nonsignificant change in favor of the control in boys and a nonsignificant change in favor of the intervention for girls (Appendix E. Evidence Table 6b).[105]

Weight

Three studies reported on weight change in the entire population. These studies showed changes in weight in favor of the control. These changes were not significant in two studies,[99,103] and the changes were significant in the other (p<0.05) (Appendix E. Evidence Table 6a).[96]

Three studies reported on weight change in subgroups, two by sex subgroups and one by grade. One study reported nonsignificant changes in weight in favor of the intervention for both boys and girls,[105] and the other showed nonsignificant changes in favor of the intervention for boys and nonsignificant changes in favor of the control for girls.[71] The third study reporting on grade subgroups reported nonsignificant changes in favor of the intervention in grades K-3 and nonsignificant changes in favor of the control for grades 4-7 (Appendix E. Evidence Table 6b).[102]

Clinical Outcomes

Seven studies reported on clinical outcomes. Five studies reported on change in systolic and diastolic blood pressure. One study reported a statistically significant change in both blood pressure measures in favor of the control (p<0.001 for both). Three of the remaining four studies reported nonsignificant changes in both blood pressure measures in favor of the intervention.[48,67,96] A single study reported a change in systolic blood pressure in favor of the intervention and a change in diastolic blood pressure in favor of the control.[91] An additional study reported on systolic and diastolic blood pressure SDS in 5 to 7 year olds, and 10 to 12 year olds. The study reported no significant difference in either measure in both groups.[63]

Six studies reported on metabolic measures. Three studies reported on HDL. One reported nonsignificant change in favor of the control.[48] Two studies reported significant changes in favor of the control, p>0.001[70], and p=0.014[100] Two studies reported on LDL changes. Both reported changes in favor of the intervention, one nonsignificant,[67] and the other significant (p<0.001)[100] Five studies reported total cholesterol. Three of these reported nonsignificant changes in favor of the control.[67,70,96] Two reported nonsignificant changes in favor of the intervention.[48,104] One reported significant changes in favor of the intervention (p<0.001).[100] A single study reported on triglycerides and showed nonsignificant changes (Appendix E. Evidence Table 6c).[100]

Adverse Events

One study[110] reported on musculoskeletal injury and used a combined intervention of diet and physical activity in a school-based setting. In year 1, there were 24 adverse events. Overall, there were 0.0006 adverse events per program hour (or incident rate 0.06 per student). Another study reported that at least one adverse event was reported by 2.4 percent of students at baseline, and 1.7 percent of students at the end of the study with no significant difference between the intervention and control groups.(Appendix E. Evidence Table 6d).[46]

Intermediate Outcomes

Physical Activity and Sedentary Behavior

Three studies measured changes in hours spent weekly in physical activity. Two studies showed no significant intervention effect.[51,72] Another study measured differences in the amount of physical activity based on where the physical activity took place.[101] In this study there was a significant difference in the weekly hours spent doing physical activity in favor of the intervention (p<0.001) inside of school, a significant difference in the weekly hours spent doing physical activity in favor of the intervention (p<0.05) outside of school, and a significant difference in the weekly hours spent doing physical activity in favor of the intervention (p<0.001) both in and outside of school.[101]

One study measured physical activity in 30 minute blocks per day and found the overall change in the amount of physical activity was not significantly different in favor of the control for groups engaged in moderate to physical activity.[50]

Seven studies, described in eight articles, measured changes in moderate to vigorous physical activity in hours per day.[56,57,60,68,75,81,100,104] Two of these showed significant increases in physical activity favoring the intervention, p=0.006,[68] p=0.04.[57] Another study reported significant change in physical activity in favor of the control at 6 years, p<0.05[104] and 10 years, p=0.038.[100] Three studies measured the change in vigorous physical activity and found no intervention effect.[60,68,81] A single study measured a physical activity index measured as sedentary activity, low activity, moderate activity, and vigorous activity.[62] All of these measures changed in favor of the intervention, but the changes were not significant.

One study measured the percentage of participants who ran in the morning or afternoon and found no difference between groups.[53] This study also found no difference in playground activity between groups. One study reported the prevalence of active commuting over time and found a significant increase in favor of the intervention.[95]

A study measured daily physical activity via accelerometer and found significant increases in the intervention group over time ($p < 0.050$).[95] Another study measured leisure time physical activity and found a significant increase in the intervention group ($p = 0.0005$).[103]

Two studies measured sedentary activity, neither found a significant difference between the intervention and control groups, but did show change in favor of the intervention.[50,62] We did not conduct meta-analyses on intermediate outcomes (Appendix E, Evidence Table 6e).

Dietary Intake

Five studies reported on the change in energy intake (e.g., caloric intake, J/day), and four reported a change in the total population in favor of the intervention, but it was not significant.[56,60,62,90] One study, reporting on the whole population, showed a significant change in energy intake in favor of the intervention ($p < 0.05$).[104] One study, reporting on sex subgroups, showed a change in energy intake in favor of the intervention in boys ($p < 0.05$), but not in girls ($p > 0.05$).[56]

Seven articles described five studies measured change in the consumption of food high in fat. Four of these studies reported data on the total population and three of these studies showed no difference in consumption between the intervention and control,[51,97] one reported a nonsignificant change in favor of the intervention,[70] one reported a nonsignificant change in favor of the control[70] A single study did show a significant difference in favor of the intervention at 6 years, $p < 0.05$.[104] One study reported on sex subgroups and found nonsignificant changes in favor of the intervention.[56] One of these studies also measured the recall of fatty food intake but found no differences between groups.[51] One paper measured energy from saturated fat and found no difference between the intervention and control (Appendix E, Evidence Table 6e).[70]

Eight studies reported on changes in fruit and vegetable intake. Two studies reported on change in vegetable intake. One did not find significant differences between intervention and control,[72] and the second showed a nonsignificant change in favor of the control.[53] A single study measured fruit intake only and found a significant increase in intake in boys (<0.05).[53] Five studies measured fruit and vegetable intake. Four of these looked at fruit and vegetable intake in the whole population. Two studies reported a nonsignificant change in intake in favor of the intervention,[50,65] one reported a nonsignificant change in favor of the control.[90] Two studies reported significant changes, both in favor of the intervention ($p = 0.003$),[56] and ($p < 0.05$).[53] One study found a significant increase among girls in the intervention group ($p = 0.003$),[56] but not in boys.

Six studies reported on sugar-sweetened beverage consumption. None showed a statistically significant change in consumption, but two studies showed a change in the direction in favor of the intervention.[50,95]

A single study[58] reported multiple measures of change in dietary intake. None of these changed significantly in this study. One study reported on change in consumption of unfavorable foods.[94] The intervention group showed a significant change in favor of the intervention ($p = 0.002$) (Appendix E, Evidence Table 6e).

41

Interpretation

The results from an outcome measure from each of the 37 studies reporting on combination diet and physical activity interventions support our conclusions. Ten studies reported on BMI z-scores.[51,55,59,62,71,72,84,85,99] Seven of these reported changes in BMI z-score in favor of the intervention,[55,59,62,71,72,84,99] with four of these reporting statistically significant changes.[62,71,84,99] Seventeen studies (described in 19 articles) reported on BMI.[47,48,50,57,58,61,65,67-69,83,88,91,98,100,103-105,111] Eleven of these studies reported a change in BMI in favor of the intervention,[48,50,57,58,65,68,88,98,100,103,104,111] with five of these reporting statistical significance.[68,88,98,100,103,104,111] Five studies reported on change in the prevalence in obesity or overweight.[53,56,64,74,90] Only one of these studies showed a change in prevalence over time in favor of the intervention, and the change was not significant.[90] Two studies reported on percentage body fat.[63,96] Neither of these studies reported a change in percentage body fat in favor of the intervention. Two studies reported on skinfold thickness.[66,70] Neither of these studies reported a change in skinfold thickness in favor of the intervention. Based on this evidence we conclude that combined diet and physical activity interventions positively impact BMI z-score and BMI. In addition to this evidence, two meta-analyses of smaller sets of studies showed significant changes in favor of the intervention for both BMI and BMI a-score (p<0.001 for both outcomes). Based on this evidence we cannot conclude that combined diet and physical activity interventions positively impact prevalence of overweight and obesity, percentage body fat, and skinfold thickness.

Some diet and physical activity combined interventions appear to be effective at reducing BMI, BMI z-score, prevalence of obesity and overweight, percent body fat, waist circumference, and skinfold thickness. Often these studies specifically targeted obesity prevention and included intensive classroom physical activity lessons led by trained teachers, moderate to vigorous physical activity sessions, nutritional education materials, and healthy diet promotion and provision. The intervention studies that had significant impact took place over a duration of 52 to 156 weeks. All of these factors may have contributed to the significant effect of the intervention on weight outcomes because a more intensive implementation of the program could have a more positive influence on the anthropometric data.

The results from these studies also suggest that schools have the opportunity to raise the physical performance of children through a higher number of physical education lessons per week.[57,68,95,100,103,104] Children who followed long-term intervention program[57,68,95,100,103,104] showed significant positive changes in physical performance, whereas children in studies of shorter intervention duration had nonsignificant results. Similarly, there were significant effects of the interventions on energy intake,[56,104] reduced consumption of sweetened beverages,[95,112] and increased fruit and vegetable intake[53,56]. Overall these results indicate intervention components and intervention dose are critical to the impact of interventions on all outcomes. Long-term intervention duration and long-term followup are vital. Future studies of this type should be of sufficient duration to enable changes in anthropometry and other secondary outcomes.

Combination diet and physical activity interventions that included psychosocial aspects to the interventions had a significant impact on obesity-prevention outcomes.[62,113] Otherwise the studies included here were very heterogeneous, and no distinct difference between effective and non-effective studies can be seen.

42

Strength of the Evidence

Weight-Related Outcomes

The strength of evidence is moderate that school-only based dietary or physical activity interventions prevent obesity or overweight in children. For both interventions the majority of studies had a moderate risk of bias and consistent direction of effect in favor of the intervention. The strength of evidence is insufficient that school-only based combination diet and physical activity interventions prevent obesity or overweight in children. We identified two low risk of bias studies and used them to evaluate the strength of evidence. These studies were inconsistent; one showed a positive effect in favor of the intervention and the other showed no effect. Additionally, the studies were imprecise (Table 5; Appendix F, Strength of Evidence Table 1).

Intermediate Outcomes

We graded multiple intermediate outcomes. The strength of evidence that diet interventions impacted energy intake (measured as change in kcal, mJ, or J per day) was insufficient. One moderate risk of bias study demonstrated no intervention effect. There was insufficient evidence that physical activity impacted energy intake since no studies reported on this outcome. The strength of evidence that combination interventions impacted change in energy intake was low. Sixty percent of the studies had a moderate risk of bias and 40 percent had a low risk of bias. While all showed a favorable impact of the intervention on the outcome, the poor risk of bias scores and low precision reduced the strength of evidence.

One diet intervention study measured change in fatty food intake. This study had a moderate risk of bias, and reported only on subgroups. A nonsignificant positive impact of the intervention in favor of the intervention was seen in girls and a significant difference was shown in favor of the boys. The lack of precision and consistency between the groups led to an insufficient grade. There was insufficient evidence that physical activity impacted fatty food intake since no studies reported on this outcome. There was a moderate strength of evidence that combination interventions positively impact this outcome in favor of the intervention; 80 percent of the studies were of a moderate risk of bias and all demonstrated an effect in favor of the intervention.

There was insufficient evidence that either diet or physical activity interventions changed fruit and vegetable intake since no studies reported on this outcome. There was moderate strength of evidence that combination outcomes positively impact fruit and vegetable intake. Most of the studies had a moderate risk of bias, and over 70 percent showed an impact in favor of the intervention.

There was insufficient evidence that either diet-only or physical activity-only interventions impacted change in sugar-sweetened intake since no studies reported on this outcome. There was moderate strength of evidence that combination outcomes positively impact sugar-sweetened beverage intake. Most of the studies had a moderate risk of bias, and all of them showed an impact in favor of the intervention.

There was insufficient evidence that diet-only interventions impacted change in physical activity since no studies reported on this outcome. Physical activity interventions have a moderate strength of evidence that the intervention positively impacts the outcome. All of these studies had a moderate risk of bias, all showed an impact in favor of the intervention, and they were precise. Combination interventions have a moderate strength of evidence that the intervention positively impacted the intervention. All of the studies had a moderate risk of bias and over 70 percent showed an impact in favor of the intervention.

There was insufficient evidence that diet or physical activity interventions impacted change in sedentary activity since no studies reported on this outcome. The single physical activity study had a moderate risk of bias with a significant change in favor of the intervention, but the study was too small (n-233) to make a conclusion. The strength of the evidence that combination interventions impact this outcome is low. All studies had a moderate risk of bias, but the direction of effect was inconsistent and there was low precision (Appendix F, Strength of Evidence Tables 2–7).

Table 5. Summary of the strength of evidence for weight-related outcomes in studies taking place in a school setting

Setting	Intervention, n	Years of Publication	Enrolled Participants	Studies With Low/Moderate/High Risk of Bias(n)	% With Favorable (Statistically Sig) Outcome	% With Favorable Outcome (Does Not Need to be Stat Sig)	Risk of Bias	Consistency	Precision	Directness	Strength of the Evidence
School	D, 2	1995–2012	1,782	0/2/0	50	100	Moderate	Consistent	Imprecise	Direct	Moderate
	PA, 15	1993–2011	10,086	0/13/2	26	73	Moderate	Consistent	Imprecise	Direct	Moderate
	C, 37	1985–2012	41,875	2/27/8	45	54	Low	Inconsistent	Imprecise	Direct	Insufficient

D = diet intervention; PA = physical activity intervention; C = combination of diet and physical activity interventions

*Total = 54-one study reported on diet, physical activity, and combination interventions, therefore was counted more than once.

45

Figure 3. Meta-analysis of change in BMI z-score between the control and combined diet and physical activity intervention groups in three school-only settings

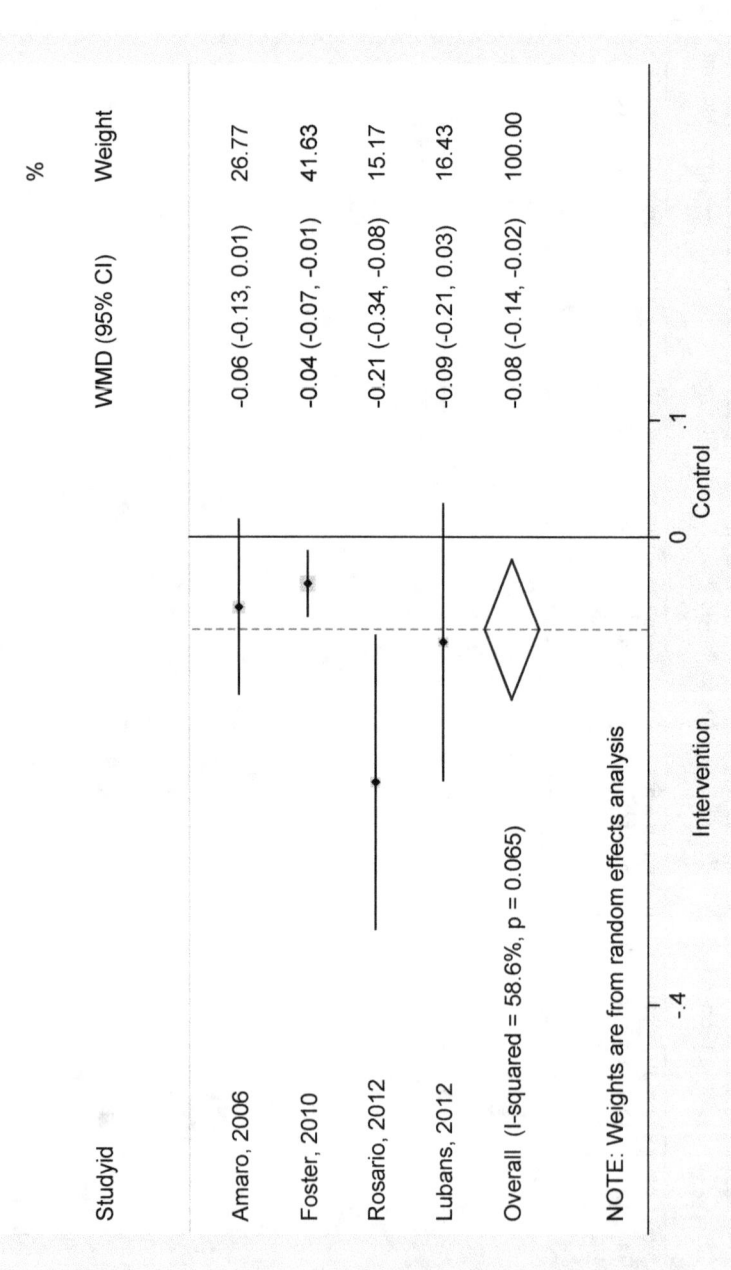

NOTE: Weights are from random effects analysis

WMD = weighted mean difference

Figure 4. Meta-analysis of change in BMI between the control and combined diet and physical activity intervention groups in four school-only settings

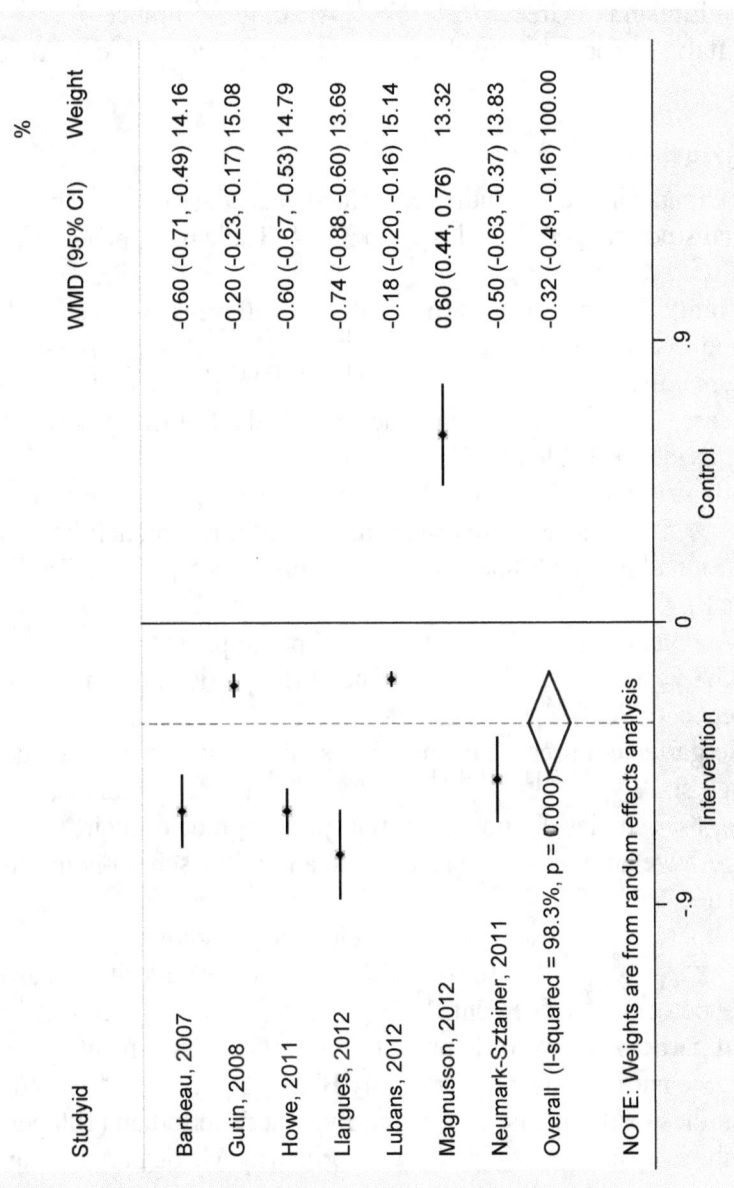

WMD = weighted mean difference

School-Home–Based Studies

Study Characteristics

Thirty studies reported on interventions delivered in the school and home settings. Of these, 21 (70 percent) were RCTs,[114-134] and 9 (30 percent) were non-RCTs.[135-143] Six of the non-RCTs consisted of a non-randomized control group design,[135-138,140,142], one was a pre-test/post-test, matched control group, quasi-experimental design[143], one was a pretest/posttest study design, [141] and one used a serial cross-sectional design.[139] Twenty-four studies (80 percent) measured obesity prevention in children.[115-117,119-123,125-133,136-139,141-143] The remaining studies measured other outcomes but contained data on weight maintenance.[114,124,134,135,140] (Table 6; Appendix E, Evidence Table 7).

Fifteen studies (48 percent) took place in the U.S.,[114-117,119,122,126,130,133,134,138,139,141-143] and the remainder were conducted in England,[129] Greece,[123,124,135,140] Australia,[118] France,[132] Germany,[120,127,131] Israel,[136] Italy,[137] Spain,[128] Sweden,[125] and Switzerland (Table 6; Appendix E, Evidence Table 7).[121]

Population Characteristics

The total number of participants in the 30 studies combined was 28,413.[114-143] The number of participants in each individual study ranged from 114[141] to 3,714 (Table 6; Appendix E, Evidence Table 8).[122]

The length of follow-up ranged from 26 weeks (6 months) to 520 weeks (10 years). Eleven studies had a follow-up period of 1 year or less.[114,116-118,121,123,127,131,137,139,140] Twelve studies had a follow-up period of between 1 and 2 years,[119,126,128-130,133,134,136,138,141-143] six studies had a follow-up period of 3 or 4 years,[115,120,122,125,132,135] and one study had a follow-up period of 10 years (Table 6; Appendix E, Evidence Table 8).[124]

All studies contained both girls and boys, and all but three studies reported the percentage of girls in the study.[114,116,117,119-136,138-143] Most studies had roughly half girls and half boys, with the percentage of girls ranging from a low of 44.8 percent[116] to a high of 58.5 percent (Table 6; Appendix E, Evidence Table 8).[130,133]

Twenty-three studies (77 percent) reported the mean age of participants,[114,115,117-121,123,125-134,138-142] which ranged from 5.8 years[126] to 13.2 years.[123] The oldest participant was 14 years old (Table 6; Appendix E, Evidence Table 8).[140]

One study included kindergarten children[126]; twenty-four studies (80 percent) included children in grades one through six.[114-117,119-122,124,125,127-136,139,141-143] one study included children in grade seven.[123] The remaining four studies did not report the specific grade of their participants.[118,137,138,140] There were no high school students in any of the school-home studies (Table 6; Appendix E, Evidence Table 8).

Thirteen of 30 studies (43 percent) reported the race or ethnicity of study participants.[114,115,119,122,126,130,133,134,138,139,141-143] In five of the studies, the majority of participants were white (63 percent,[119] 69 percent,[122] 78 percent,[142] 83 percent,[134] and 94 percent).[141] In three of the studies, the majority of participants were Hispanic (66 percent,[139] 68 percent,[138] and 93 per).[143] In two of the studies, the participants were primarily Black (68 percent[130] and 46 percent)[133]; in another two studies, participants were primarily American Indian (100 percent[126] and ≥ 90 percent[115]); and in the last study, participants were primarily Mexican American (80 percent).[114] Among the studies that did not report race, only two were U.S. studies.[116,117] (Table 6; Appendix E, Evidence Table 8).

Interventions

Twenty-six of the 30 studies (87 percent) included combined diet and physical activity interventions.[114-116,118-120,122-131,133-136,138-143] (Table 7; Appendix E, Evidence Table 9). One study included an intervention that focused exclusively on diet modification.[137] (Table 7; Appendix E, Evidence Table 9). Two studies focused exclusively on physical activity interventions,[121,132] and a third study focused on the reduction of sedentary behavior associated with television, videotape, and videogame use (Table 7; Appendix E, Evidence Table 9).[117] There were no studies that reported on self-management alone (Table 7; Appendix E, Evidence Table 9).

Table 6. Study and participant characteristics of studies based in schools with a home component

Author, Year	RCT	Goal: Weight Maint	Country	Sex*	Age Range, Years*	Grade*	Other*	Total N	Followup in Weeks	% Girls†	Mean Age [Range] Years†	Grade†	Race†
Brandstetter, 2012[127]	Y	Y	Germany	NR	NR	2	NR	1119	52	46.3%	7.57	2	NR
Burke, 1998[118]	Y	N	Australia	NR	NR	NR	NR	800	26	49%	11	NR	NR
Caballero, 2003[115]	Y	Y	U.S	NR	NR	3	NR	1,704	156	NR	7.6	3	≥ 90% American Indian
Coleman, 2005[143]	N	Y	U.S	NR	NR	NR	NR	896	104	47.2%	NR	3	93% Hispanic
Danielzik, 2007[120]	Y	Y	Germany	NR	NR	NR	NR	1,764	208	50.5%	6.3	1	NR
Dzewaltowski, 2010[119]	Y	Y	U.S	NR	NR	NR	NR	273	104	50%	9.3	3,4	62.7% WNH, 18.8% BNH, 8.9% American Indian, 6.6% Hispanic, 3% Other
Foster, 2008[133]	Y	Y	U.S	NR	NR	NR	NR	1,349	104	53.7%	11.2	4, 5, 6	45.6% BNH, 22.4% Asian, 14.1% Hispanic, 12.4% WNH, 5.5% Other
Hatzis, 2010[124]	Y	N	Greece	NR	NR	NR	NR	634	520	52.4%	NR	1	NR
Hendy, 2011[116]	Y	Y	U.S	NR	NR	NR	NR	382	52	44.8%	NR	1,2,3,4	NR
Hoelscher, 2010[139]	N	Y	U.S	NR	NR	NR	NR	1,107	52	53%	9.9	4	66% Hispanic, 20% WNH, 14% BNH

Table 6. Study and participant characteristics of studies based in schools with a home component (continued)

Author, Year	RCT	Goal: Weight Maint	Country	Sex*	Age Range, Years*	Grade*	Other*	Total N	Followup in Weeks	% Girls†	Mean Age [Range] Years†	Grade†	Race†
Hollar, 2010[138]	N	Y	U.S	NR	NR	NR	NR	1,197	68	51%	7.8	NR	68% Hispanic, 15% WNH, 9% BNH, 8% Other
Hopper, 2005[134]	Y	N	U.S	NR	NR	NR	NR	238	86	49%	7.6	3	83% WNH, 5% Hispanic, 5% Asian, 5% American Indian, 2% BNH
Kriemler, 2010[121]	Y	Y	Switzerland	NR	NR	NR	NR	502	47	51%	6.9, 11.1	1,5	NR
Llargues, 2011[128]	Y	Y	Spain	NR	NR	1st year primary school	NR	509	76	45.9%	6.03	1	NR
Lloyd, 2012[129]	Y	Y	England	NR	9-10 years old	Year 5 class	NR	202	72-96 weeks	50.0%	9.69	5	NR
Lionis, 1991[140]	N	N	Greece	NR	13-14	NR	NR	171	39	51%	13-14	NR	NR
Manios, 1998[135]	N	N	Greece	NR	NR	NR	NR	962	156	47%	NR	1	NR
Marcus, 2009[125]	Y	Y	Sweden	NR	NR	NR	NR	3,152	208	49%	7.5	1,2,3,4	NR
Mihas, 2010[123]	Y	Y	Greece	NR	12-13	7	NR	191	52	49%	13.2	7	NR
Nader, 1999[122]	Y	Y	U.S	NR	NR	NR	NR	3,714	156	48%	NR	3	69% WNH, 14% Hispanic, 13% BNH, 4% Other
Robinson, 1999[117]	Y	Y	U.S	NR	NR	3, 4	NR	198	26	46.6%	8.9	3, 4	NR
Schetzina, 2009[141]	N	Y	U.S	NR	NR	NR	NR	114	78	53%	9	3, 4	94% WNH, 3% BNH, 3% Other
Shofan, 2011[136]	N	Y	Israel	NR	NR	NR	NR	118	104	46.6%	9-11	4,5,6	NR

Table 6. Study and participant characteristics of studies based in schools with a home component (continued)

Author, Year	RCT	Goal: Weight Maint	Country	Sex*	Age Range, Years*	Grade*	Other*	Total N	Followup in Weeks	% Girls[†]	Mean Age [Range] Years[†]	Grade[†]	Race[†]
Siegrist, 2011[131]	Y	N/NR	Germany	NR	NR	2 and 3	NR	724	52	48.3%	8.4	2,3	NR
Simon, 2008[132]	Y	Y	France	NR	NR	NR	NR	954	208	50.0%	11.6	6	NR
Simonetti D'Arca, 1986[137]	N	Y	Italy	NR	NR	NR	NR	1,321	52	NR	3-9	NR	NR
Speroni, 2007[142]	N	Y	U.S	NR	NR	NR	NR	185	104	50.3%	9.3	2, 4	78.3% WNH, 21.7% Hispanic
Story, 2012[126]	Y	Y	U.S.	NR	NR	Kinder-garten	NR	454	80	48.9%	5.81	Kinder-garten	100% American Indian
Trevino, 2004[114]	Y	N	U.S	NR	<12	4	NR	1,419	34	49.5%	9.8	4	80% Mexican American
Williamson, 2012[130]	Y	Y	U.S.	NR	NR	4 to 6; rural commun ities	NR	2060	121	58.5%	10.5	4,5,6	31.6% WNH; 68.4% Black

AIAN = American Indian/Alaska Native; API = Asian Pacific Islander; BMI = Body Mass Index (in kg/m²); BNH = Black Non-Hispanic; BP = Blood Pressure; CVD = Cardio Vascular Disease.; Maint = Maintenance; Meds = Medications; N = No; NR = Not Reported; physical activity = Physical Activity; RCT = Randomized Controlled Trials; WNH = White Non-Hispanic; Y=Yes

*Inclusion/exclusion criteria.
[†]Participant characteristics.

52

Table 7. Interventions of studies based in schools with a home component

Author, Year	Control Arm	Description of Intervention	Diet (Phys/Env)	Diet (Psych)	Physical Activity (Phys/Env)	Physical Activity (Psych)
Brandstetter, 2012[127]	Usual care	URMEL-ICE: School health promoting behavior change Family homework lessons, training and information of parents.	X		X	X
Burke, 1998[118]	Usual care	WASPAN[a] Classroom lessons on physical activity and nutrition. Home-based nutritional program for children and their families.	X			X
	Usual care	WASPAN[b] Classroom nutrition and physical activity lessons with physical education enrichment activities. Home-based nutritional program for children and family.	X			X
Caballero, 2003[115]	Usual care	Classroom curriculum Family involvement.	X	X	X	X
Coleman, 2005[143]	Usual care	Classroom and school wide physical education and nutrition changes in the cafeteria Home reduction of sedentary activity	X	X	X	X
Danielzik, 2007[120]	Usual care	Behavioral and educational messages using nutrition fairy tales about eating fruit and vegetables every day and reduce intake of high-fat foods. Behavioral and educational messages to keep active and decrease television consumption Preparing a healthy breakfast at home	X		X	
Dzewaltowski, 2010[119]	Usual care	HOP'N after school: a weekly social-cognitive-theory based curriculum (eat fruits and vegetables and increase physical activity). Home—no more than 2 hours a day sedentary activity; remove TV from the bedroom.	X	X	X	X
Foster, 2008[133]	Usual care	School Nutrition Policy Initiative: classroom-based nutrition education, foods sold met a specified nutritional standard; physical activity linked to personal behavior. Reduced sedentary activity at home.	X	X	X	
Gorely, 2009[144]	Usual care	GreatFun2Run: increase children's activities through physical activity on running. Raise awareness at home	X		X	X
Hatzis, 2010[124]	Usual care	"Know Your Body" education material with major modifications to the Mediterranean diet of Crete and the orthodox Christian church fasting rituals.	X		X	
Hendy, 2011[116]	Usual care	KCP group (LIONS)-received stars for 3 good health behaviors.	X		X	

53

Table 7. Interventions of studies based in schools with a home component (continued)

Author, Year	Control Arm	Description of Intervention	Diet (Phys/Env)	Diet (Psych)	Physical Activity (Phys/Env)	Physical Activity (Psych)
Hoelscher, 2010[139]	Usual care	CATCH BP[c] Classroom curricula and a physical education program, a child nutrition services component Family involvement	X	X	X	X
	Usual care	CATCH BPC[d] Classroom curricula and a physical education program, a child nutrition services component Family involvement Community action team	X	X	X	X
Hollar, 2010[138]	Usual care	HOPS intervention: School provided diet, classroom curricula, and physical activity during school day.	X	X	X	X
Hopper, 2005[134]	Usual care	School classroom lessons on nutrition and exercise. Home activities for parents and children to complete.	X		X	X
Kriemler, 2010[121]	Usual care	KISS: School based stringent physical activity program Home daily physical activity homework of about 10 minutes.				X
Lionis, 1991[140]	Usual care	School health education curriculum.	X		X	
Llargues, 2011[128]	Usual care	Education about food habits and physical activity: developing posters, food tables, games, crafts, cooking workshops and promotion of games in the playground.	X		X	
Lloyd, 2012[129]	Usual care	School newsletters, plays, homework, assembly Home: multiple activities involving home and parents	X		X	
Manios, 1998[135]	Usual care	School health education plus physical activity components. Provide parents screening results and lessons on the importance of children's dietary and exercise habits.	X		X	X
Marcus, 2009[125]	Usual care	Diet and physical activity awareness: Change the school environment, including school lunches, afternoon snacks, after school care activities and sports days. Parents were asked not to provide unhealthy snacks for birthdays etc.		X	X	X
Mihas, 2010[123]	Usual care	Health and nutrition education	X		X	
Nader, 1999[122]	Usual care	CATCH intervention: targeted consuming foods low in fat, saturated fat and sodium via a multicomponent program that included school environmental changes, and a family component.	X	X	X	X
Robinson, 1999[117]	Usual care	Classroom curriculum to reduce television, videotape, and video game use.			X	X

54

Table 7. Interventions of studies based in schools with a home component (continued)

Author, Year	Control Arm	Description of Intervention	Diet (Phys/Env)	Diet (Psych)	Physical Activity (Phys/Env)	Physical Activity (Psych)
Schetzina, 2009[141]	Usual care	Winning with Wellness Pilot program: classroom instruction, school health services, and removing soda from vending machines and physical education and activity	X		X	X
Shofan, 2011[136]	Usual care	Focused on increased physical education and activity together with nutritional advice to the children and their families.	X			X
Siegrist, 2011[131]	Usual care	JuvenTUM: educate students, parents and teachers; alter school environments for diet and physical activity	X	X	X	X
Simon, 2008[132]	Usual care	School education on physical activity and sedentary behaviors, opportunities for physical activity were offered. Parents were asked to support the child's physical activity.			X	X
Simonetti D'Arca, 1986[137]	Usual care	Written Action School: Focused on educating staff, students and parents using printed material only.	X			
	Usual care	Multi-media Action School: Focused on educating staff, students and parents using media.	X			
Speroni, 2007[142]	Usual care	After-school exercise and diet education program	X			X
Story, 2012[126]	Usual care	Bright Start: School physical activity sessions, nutritional lessons Goal to increase health awareness and better eating habits at home through motivational interventions		X		X
Trevino, 2004[114]	Usual care	School health behavior messages in classroom, school cafeteria, and after-school care. Reinforced at home and after school care.	X		X	X
Williamson, 2012[130]	Usual care	School change in food from school cafeterias and vending machines, physical activity in class, during recess and PE classes Newsletters sent home providing campaign-specific information		X		X

Phys/Env = Physical/environmental intervention; Psych = psychosocial intervention
[a]Western Australian Schools Physical Activity and Nutrition.
[b]Western Australian Schools Physical Activity and Nutrition plus physical activity enrichment for children with high cardiovascular risk.
[c]Coordinated Approach To Child Health BasicPlus (CATCH BP).
[d]Coordinated Approach To Child Health BasicPlus (CATCH BP) plus Community.

55

Outcomes

Diet Interventions

There was one diet-only intervention, which employed an educational approach to diet and nutrition (Appendix E, Evidence Table 10a,b).[137]

Weight-Related Outcomes

Prevalence of Overweight and Obesity

This RCT with 1,321 participants [137] measured the change of prevalence in overweight and obesity after 1 year. It compared two different interventions to one control group. In the control school, students received usual care. The study called one intervention the written action (WA) intervention, and the other the multi-media action (MA) intervention. The results of this study demonstrated an increase in the prevalence of overweight students (+0.8 percent) and obese students (+5.9 percent) in the control group. The WA intervention arm led to a 2.3 percent decrease in overweight students, but a 5.3 percent increase in obese students. However, the MA intervention led to 12.1 percent reduction in the prevalence of overweight students and a 12.2 percent reduction in the prevalence of obese students at the end of the study.(Appendix E, Evidence Table 10a,b).

Among boys, there was a 2.0 percent reduction in overweight in the control group versus the MA group, and a 1.6 percent increase in the control group versus the WA group. Among girls, there was a 5.4 percent reduction in overweight in the control group versus the MA group, and a 3.7 percent reduction in the control group versus the WA group (Appendix E, Evidence Table 10a). Among boys, there was a 2.6 percent reduction in obese children in the control group versus the MA group, and a 1.1 percent increase in the control group versus the WA group. Among girls, there was a 2.2 percent reduction in obese children in the control group versus the MA group, and a 1.0 percent increase in the control group versus the WA group (Appendix E, Evidence Table 10a).

Clinical Outcomes

The research did not report any.

Adverse Events

The research did not report any.

Intermediate Outcomes

The research did not report any.

Interpretation

The results from an outcome measure from this study support our conclusions. In this study, the less intensive intervention, which relied exclusively on the dissemination of printed material, was less effective in reducing the prevalence of overweight and obesity compared to the intervention, which employed qualified staff to interact directly with students, teachers, and parents through meetings, discussions, and other interactive activities.

Physical Activity Interventions

Two studies focused exclusively on physical activity interventions. These studies were multi-component physical activity programs that included both an educational and environmental approach to physical activity.[121,132] A third study focused on the reduction of sedentary behavior associated with television, videotape, and videogame use (Appendix E, Evidence Table 11a,b).[117]

Weight-Related Outcomes

BMI

Of the three studies reported above that measured change in BMI,[121,132,117] all three showed a statistically significant reduction in the intervention group relative to the control group: -0.12 (p<.003); -0.26 at 2 years, -0.25 at 3 years, and -0.25 at 4 years, (p=0.01), and -0.45 (p=.002), respectively (Appendix E, Evidence Table 11a,b).

Prevalence of Overweight and Obesity

One physical activity study found a reduction in the prevalence of overweight in the intervention group relative to the control: at 4 years; 4.2 percent of the initially non-overweight students were overweight in the intervention schools, compared to 9.8 percent in the control schools (odds ratio [OR], 95% confidence interval [CI]=0.41 [0.22; 0.75]) (Appendix E, Evidence Table 11a,b).[132]

Percent Body Fat

One study stratified the analysis according to "initially non-overweight" and "initially overweight" participants, the results showed an improvement in percent body fat in the "initially non-overweight" group (-0.55 percent, p=0.19) in the intervention group, but a worsening in the "initially overweight" group (1.33 percent, p=0.18) (Appendix E, Evidence Table 11a,b).[132]

Waist Circumference

Of the two studies that measured change in waist circumference (cm),[121,117] both showed a reduction in waist circumference in the intervention group relative to the control group, -0.08 (p=0.25) and -2.30 (p<0.001), respectively (Appendix E, Evidence Table 11a,b).

Skinfold Thickness

The study that measured triceps skinfold thickness showed a decrease of 1.47 (p=0.002) in the intervention group relative to the control group (Appendix E, Evidence Table 11 a,b).[117]

The study that measured change in the sum of four skinfolds showed an decrease of 0.12 (p=0.009) in the intervention group relative to the control group (Appendix E, Evidence Table 11a,b).[121]

Clinical Outcomes

One study computed a cardiovascular risk score that included all components of the metabolic syndrome, including average z-score of waist circumference, mean blood pressure, blood glucose, inverted HDL cholesterol, and triglycerides. The results showed that the intervention resulted in an improvement in the cardiovascular risk score, corresponding to 0.18 (−0.29 to −0.06) z-score units (p=0.003).[121] Two studies found a reduction of -0.08 mm Hg (p=0.88)[121] and -0.42 mm Hg (p=0.66)[132] in systolic blood pressure in favor of the intervention, but neither result was statistically significant. Two studies[121][132] found a reduction of 0.12 (p=0.02) and 0.46 (p=0.60), respectively in diastolic blood pressure, mostly in favor of the intervention relative to the control group. One study found an increase in total cholesterol of 2.71 (p=0.15) in the intervention group relative to the control group.[132] Two studies showed an increase in HDL. One showed an increase in HDL of 3.43 (p<0.0001),[132] and one showed a decrease of -0.78 which was not significant.[140] Two studies[121][132] found a reduction in triglycerides in favor of the intervention (-0.10, p<0.02) and (-2.60, p=0.34), respectively. One study[132] found no difference in glucose between the intervention and control group (0.0, p=0.81). One study found a slight increase in the intervention group relative to the control group (0.03 (95% CI -0.98; 1.04) p=0.96), and a slight increase in HOMA in the intervention group relative to the control group (0.01 (95% CI -0.23; 0.24) p=0.95) (Appendix E, Evidence Table 11c).[132]

Adverse Events

The research did not report any.

Intermediate Outcomes

One study reported a large number of intermediate outcomes which included a series of child and parent reported measures of television viewing, diet, and physical activity and fitness.[117] The children-reported measures showed a consistent reduction (on a per-week basis) in favor of the intervention group with respect to all of the following measures: 5.53 fewer hours of television (p<0.001), 1.53 fewer hours of videotapes (p=0.11), 2.54 fewer hours of videogame usage (p=0.01), 0.54 fewer meals in front of the TV (p=0.01), 0.11 fewer snacks in front of the television (p=0.16), 0.82 fewer daily servings of high fat food (p=0.12), and 0.34 fewer other sedentary behaviors (p=0.44). The only outcomes that did not show a reduction were daily servings of high-advertised foods (increase of 0.06, p=0.71) and the 20-meter shuttle test (fewer cones by 0.87, p=0.45).[117]

Parent reports of their children's behavior yielded similar results: 4.29 fewer hours of TV (p<0.001), 0.25 fewer hours of videotapes (p=0.60), 0.76 fewer video game hours (p=0.13), 0.77 fewer hours of household TV use (p=0.10), 1.1 fewer meals in front of the TV (p=0.02), 1.9 percentage decline in TV viewing while snacking (p=0.59), 4.88 fewer other sedentary behaviors (p=0.16), and 2.0 more hours/week of physical activity, (p=0.13) (Appendix E, Evidence Table 11d).[117]

In another study, there was an improvement in the Shuttle Run of 0.17 cones in the intervention group relative to the control group (p=0.04); an increase in in-school physical activity (counts/min) by 0.92 (p=0.003); and an increase in in-school total moderate to vigorous physical activity (min/day) by 1.19, p<0.001.[121] In a second study, intervention students had an increase in supervised physical activity (p=0.0001) and a reduction in TV/video viewing (p=0.01) relative to the control group (Appendix E, Evidence Table 11d).[132]

Interpretation

The results from an outcome measure from these two studies support our conclusions. Even though two of the three studies focused on increasing physical activity and the other focused on decreasing sedentary behavior, they all demonstrated some improvements in BMI, waist circumference, and skinfold thickness due to the intervention. This suggests that interventions aimed at either increasing physical activity or reducing sedentary behavior can be effective at preventing obesity.

Diet and Physical Activity Interventions

Twenty-six of 30 studies conducted in both the school and home setting implemented combined diet and physical activity interventions. Of the 27, 18 were RCTs (Appendix E, Evidence Table 12a,b).

Weight-Related Outcomes

Twenty-three out of 30 studies included a measure of BMI, BMI z-score, or BMI percentile. Of these, six were statistically significant in favor of the intervention, 14 were nonsignificant, two did not report p-values, and one had inconsistent results.

BMI z-Score

Among the eight studies that measured BMI z-score, one showed significant reductions in favor of the intervention (-0.34)[138,144] and the rest did not.[120,126,129-131,133,141]

BMI

Among the 17 studies that measured BMI, 14 showed a reduction in BMI in the intervention group relative to the control group, with the magnitude of difference ranging from -0.4 to -1.20 kg/m^2. However, only four of these changes were statistically significant. [124,128,135,140]

There were seven studies[118,119,126,131] (but a total of eight active intervention arms) that we included in a meta-analysis for the BMI (kg/m^2) outcome measure. The results of the meta-analysis yielded an overall weighted mean difference of 95 percent -0.17 kg/m^2 (95% CI: -0.57, 0.23, p=0.407), which favored the control over the intervention, but was not statistically significant. Studies were excluded from the meta-analysis for the following reasons: a) if they were not an RCT, b) if there was considerable heterogeneity when included in the analysis, c) if there was insufficient outcome reporting, or d) if there was an insufficient numbers of studies with a similar intervention. (Figure 5) (Appendix E, Evidence Table 12 a, b).

One study compared one control arm with two intervention arms.[118] One intervention arm was the Western Australian Schools Physical Activity and Nutrition project, and the second intervention arm was Western Australian Schools Physical Activity and Nutrition project plus a physical education enrichment program targeting only children with higher levels of cardiovascular risk (Appendix E, Evidence Table 12a). There was no improvement in BMI in either boys or girls due to either intervention arm.

BMI Percentile

Two studies reported BMI percentile. One showed a clear reduction in due to the intervention,[142] (-3.8 percent, p<0.01). The other study examined change in BMI percentile in two strata of participants: average weight participants (n=200) and overweight participants (n=112).[116] At the 3-month followup period, the results showed a nonsignificant reduction in average weight participants by 2.40 percent (p=0.32) relative to the control group, but a significant reduction in overweight participants by 2.60 percent (p=0.001). However, this reduction was not maintained when reexamined 6 months later. The third study showed no effect of the intervention on the BMI percentile.[94] (Appendix E, Evidence Table 12a,b).

Prevalence of Overweight and Obesity

Only one study examined the change in the incidence of overweight and obesity due to the intervention.[133] After controlling for gender, race/ethnicity, and age, this study found that the odds of becoming *overweight* in the intervention group were 33 percent lower for the intervention group compared to the control group (adjusted OR, 0.67 [95% CI 0.47–0.96], p<0.03). However, there were no differences in the incidence of obesity between the intervention and controls schools (adjusted OR, 1.00 [95% CI 0.66–1.52], p=0.99) (Appendix E, Evidence Table 12a,b).

After 2 years, the unadjusted prevalence of overweight had decreased by 10.3 percent in intervention schools and had increased by 25.9 percent in control schools. After controlling for gender, race/ethnicity, age, and baseline prevalence, the predicted odds of overweight prevalence were 35 percent lower for the intervention group (adjusted OR 0.65 (95% CI 0.54–0.79), p<0.0001). Similar to the results for incidence of obesity, there was no apparent reduction in the prevalence of obesity as a result of the intervention (adjusted OR 1.09 (95% CI 0.85–1.40), p=0.48) (Appendix E, Evidence Table 12a,b).

A study with similar results[126]showed a 10 percent reduction in the prevalence of overweight (between 85 and 95 percentile) in favor of the intervention group (p=0.019), but no corresponding change in the prevalence of obesity (BMI $\geq$ 95th percentile).

Another study[125] found a significant reduction in the prevalence of overweight (-3.70 percent, p<0.05), obesity (-2.30 percent, p<0.05), and the two together (-6.00 percent, p<0.05) due to the intervention (Appendix E, Evidence Table 12a,b).

One study compared two different intervention arms: the Combined Approach to Child Health (CATCH) curriculum Basic Plus (BP) and the CATCH Basic Plus Community (BPC).[139] There was no control group in this study. The CATCH BP led to a reduction of 3.1 percent (p=0.33) prevalence of overweight and obesity from baseline to followup, and the CATCH BPC led to a reduction of 8.30 percent (p<0.005), indicating that the enhance CATCH BPC had a greater effect on weight control than the CATCH BP intervention (Appendix E, Evidence Table 12a,b).

In one study, the prevalence of overweight and obesity had decreased by -7.6 percent in the intervention group by 18 months, and by -9.7 percent by 24 months.[129]

In another study, the prevalence of overweight increased by 8.0 percent in the control group but only by 5.3 percent in the intervention group, and the prevalence of obesity increased by 0.5 percent in the control group, but decreased by 3.6 percent in the intervention group. Prevalence of excess weight (overweight and obesity) increased by 8.5 percent in the control group and by 1.8 percent in the intervention group.[128]

One study that compared the risk of overweight or overweight in girls and boys found that the rate of increase in percent overweight was 2.0 percent for girls in the intervention schools compared to 13.0 percent for girls in the control schools; and 1.0 percent in boys in the intervention schools compared to 9.0 percent in the control schools (Appendix E, Evidence Table 12b).[143]

Percent Body Fat

Among the four studies that investigated change in percent body fat, only one showed a reduction in percent body fat in the intervention group relative to the control group by -0.83 at 18 months and -1.28 at 24 months.[129]; the other four demonstrated a trend in favor of the control group,[114,115,124,126] although the results were not statistically significant (Appendix E, Evidence Table 12a,b). A final study found no differences between groups in percent body fat for either girls or boys.[130]

Waist Circumference

Among the six studies that reported waist circumference, five showed a reduction due to the intervention[120,124,127,129,131](-0.80, -0.70, -0.61, -2.01, and -1,70 cm, respectively), and one study showed an increase, but the change was not significant[118] (Appendix E, Evidence Table 12a,b).

Skinfold Thickness

Among the six studies that measured change in triceps skinfold thickness, three showed an improvement in the intervention group, relative to the control group[122,127,135], and the remaining three studies revealed an increase in the intervention group, although none of these differences were statistically significant[115,122,126,140](Appendix E, Evidence Table 12a,b). Four studies measured change in subscapular skinfolds. None showed a significant difference between groups (Appendix E, Evidence Table 12a, b).[115,122,126,135]

Clinical Outcomes

One study found a small reduction in systolic blood pressure and a reduction of -2.47 mm Hg and -2.09 mm Hg, respectively in diastolic blood pressure (fourth and fifth phase) in favor of the intervention group. (Appendix E, Evidence Table 12c)[140] This study also demonstrated significant improvements in cholesterol levels in the intervention group, including a decrease in total cholesterol of -17.21 ($p<0.001$); a reduction in LDL of 17.6 (mg/l) ($p<0.0001$), and improvements in the ratio of LDL/HDL and the ratio of total cholesterol to HDL of 0.31 ($p<0.001$) and 0.31 ($p<0.001$), respectively.[140] (Appendix E, Evidence Table 12c).

Adverse Events

The research did not report any.

Intermediate Outcomes

Physical Activity and Sedentary Behavior

Fifteen of the 16 studies that measured change in physical activity showed some improvement in physical activity in the intervention group relative to the control group.

Among the studies that measured number of steps, one study demonstrated that the intervention group increased the number of steps it took by 11,971 steps per month, compared to 758 steps in the control group ($p=0.011$) (Appendix E, Evidence Table 12d).[116] In a study with a pre-test/post-test design, participants took an average of 886 more steps after the intervention compared to before ($p<0.001$).[141]

Among studies that measured total physical activity, one study showed a slight increase in total physical activity of 0.30 hours/wk (95 percent CI- 0.40 to 1.0 hr/wk, $p=0.40$) and a corresponding reduction in total inactivity in the intervention group relative to the control ($p<0.001$) (Appendix E, Evidence Table 12).[133] Another study demonstrated a 10.8 percent increase in the proportion of students who exercised greater than or equal to 7 times per week, but no increase in the actual exercise intensity (-0.30). One study showed that participants in the intervention group increased the amount of time they spent playing outside (by 2 percent), participating in sports clubs (by 5 percent) and participating in sport activity outside of sports club (by 8 percent) compared to the control group.[127] Another study showed an increase of 10 percent in the intervention group in the amount of physical activity performed outside of school compared to the control group.[145] Two other studies showed an increase in the number of active days per week[131] and the number of minutes of physical activity per week[126], but neither of these results were statistically significant. One study demonstrated an improvement in physical activity in three out of five measures, including number of days engaged in at least 30 minutes of vigorous physical activity (0.3), number of days played outdoors (0.1), and number of days played sports activity (0.2); but there was no improvement in the percent engaged in at least 30 minutes of vigorous physical activity per day (-0.6), nor in the number of days participated in some organized activity (-0.1) (Appendix E, Evidence Table 12d).[139]

Among studies that measured moderate to vigorous physical activity, one study showed a statistically significant improvement of 1.6 minutes ($p<0.005$) in the intervention group relative to the control group. (Appendix E, Evidence Table 12d).[135] Another study demonstrated a 3 percent increase in the number of students engaged in vigorous physical activity ($p<0.05$) and a 5 percent increase in the number of students engaged in moderate to vigorous physical activity (nonsignificant) in the intervention group relative to the control group (Appendix E, Evidence Table 12d).[143] A final study showed an improvement of 8.8 more minutes of vigorous physical activity in the intervention compared to the control group ($p=0.001$) (Appendix E, Evidence Table 12d).[122]

In one study, there was a nonsignificant increase in physical activity according to a motion sensor (average vector magnitude/min) of 20.43 (95% CI= -19.05, 59.92) in the intervention group relative to the control group ($p=0.310$) (Appendix E, Evidence Table 12).[115] And another study showed an increase of 18 counts per minute of physical activity in the intervention group compared to the control group. The one study that did not show improvement measured physical activity by a self-administered activity checklist.[130]

Seven studies measured change in sedentary behavior. All five of the studies that measured screen time, showed a reduction in TV, video, or computer usage in the intervention group compared to the control group.[118,127,129,133,139] In one study, which compared the CATCH BP Program to CATCH BPC, the BPC group showed a 4.7 percent reduction ($p=0.095$) among students who watched greater than 2 hours of TV per day, a -5.6 percent reduction ($p=0.182$) among students who spent greater than 2 hours on the computer per day, and a 1.3 percent reduction ($p=0.182$) among students who played greater than 2 hours of video games per day.[139] In another study, according to student's diaries, there was no overall change in physical activity or TV-watching, except for the subgroup of boys in the physical activity enrichment arm of the study.[118] In a third study, there was a decrease in total TV hours during the weekdays by 5 percent ($p<0.0001$) and on the weekends to a lesser degree (3 percent, $p=0.39$).[133] Two other studies showed a reduction in general sedentary behavior in the intervention group compared to the control.[128,130] (Appendix E, Evidence Table 12d)

Dietary Intake

Seven of nine studies showed a reduction in caloric intake in the intervention group relative to the control.[122,123,126,130,133,134,140] Of the remaining two studies, one showed an increase in caloric intake in the intervention group,[124,134,140] and one reported a reduction of -265 (kcal) (95% CI -437 to -94, $p=0.003$) in the intervention group using a 24-hour dietary recall method, but a minor increase in caloric intake according to school-lunch observation measure. (Appendix E, Evidence Table 12d).[115]

Among the seven studies that measured change in fruit and vegetable intake, four showed improvements,[116,126,128,139] two showed no improvement,[125,133] and one showed an improvement in fruit, but not vegetable, intake due to the intervention.[123]

In the first study, the intervention group increased their fruits and vegetables first behavior by 2.31 meals (of six meals), compared to 0.72 in the control group (p=0.000) and increased their healthy drinks behavior by 3.46 meals compared to 0.52 meals in the control group, (p=0.000).[116] In the second study, there was a small improvement in the number of fruits and vegetables consumed in the intervention group (0.3, p=0.074).[139] In the third study, there was no between-group difference in the portions of vegetables consumed per week, but there was a slight, nonsignificant increase of 1.0 portion of fruit consumed per week by the intervention group relative to the control group.[123] In a fourth study, children in the intervention group reported less consumption of high-fat dairy products (p=0.001), sweetened cereals (p=0.02), and sweet products (p=0.002) than children in the control group; however, there was no between-group difference in the amount of fruits and vegetables consumed (p=0.47).[125] In the fifth study, fruit and vegetable intake decreased in both groups over time[133] (Appendix E, Evidence Table 12d).

There were four studies that showed modest improvements in the intervention group relative to the control group.[126-128,139] (Appendix E, Evidence Table 12d).[139]

There were two studies that measured change in fatty food intake. One study showed a reduction in grams of fat, percentage of total fat calories, and percentage of calories from saturated fat in the intervention group compared to the control group, however there was no change in the amount of fast food per day.[126] The other study showed a reduction on total fat and saturated fat, but these changes were not significant.[130] An additional study measured change in fatty food intake by the Unhealthy Food Index. This study demonstrated a modest, but significant decrease of -0.6 points on the Unhealthy Food index in the intervention group relative to the control (Appendix E, Evidence Table 12d).[139]

Interpretation

Our conclusions are based on one outcome measure from each of the 26 studies reporting on combined diet and physical activity interventions. Overall the findings suggest that combined diet and physical activity interventions have favorable effects on weight outcomes, as well as for increasing physical activity, reducing sedentary behavior, and promoting healthier eating.

Seventeen studies reported on BMI (kg/m^2).[115,118-120,122-124,126-129,131,133-136,140] Fourteen of these studies reported changes in favor of the intervention.[115,119,120,122-124,127-129,131,133-135,140] Among the 14, four were statistically significant.[124,128,135,140]

Two studies reported on BMI percentile,[116,142] which were statistically significant in favor of the intervention.

Three studies reported on BMI percentile,[94,116,142] and two of these were statistically significant in favor of the intervention.

Three studies reported on prevalence of overweight or obesity.[125,139,143] All three showed a significant effect in favor of the intervention.

One study reported on percent body fat.[114] This study was not in favor of the intervention, nor was it statistically significant.

The differences between the statistically significant and non-significant studies that tested a combination physical activity and diet intervention or physical activity intervention do not appear to be related to characteristics related to study participants (sex or age), type of intervention (education or environment), or country. The factors that could contribute to more successful interventions could be related to implementation; other characteristics of the intervention such as intensity, dose, and duration; and participant engagement. These types of characteristics were sought but rarely reported in studies; we were thus unable to explore the impact of these factors on our conclusions. In addition, worth noting it is possible and even likely

63

that the dose of the home component of many school-based interventions with a home component would be very low, rendering them similar to those school-only based interventions.

Since few studies included clinical outcomes, there is insufficient evidence about the impact of these types of interventions on markers of cardiovascular health.

However, many studies included measures of physical activity, sedentary behavior and dietary intake. Overall, 15 out of 16 studies showed some improvement in physical activity due to the intervention. All seven of the studies that aimed to reduce sedentary behavior, showed a reduction in TV, video, or computer use or other sedentary activity, due to the intervention. Dietary outcomes also showed improvements of various kinds: seven of nine studies showed a reduction in caloric intake in the intervention group relative to the control; four of seven studies showed an increase in fruit and vegetable intake; four of four studies showed a modest decrease in sugar-sweetened beverage intake, and two other studies demonstrated a decrease in fatty food intake.

Strength of the Evidence

Weight-Related Outcomes

The strength of the evidence is insufficient that diet interventions positively impact obesity prevention, because there is only one study that contained a diet intervention. In contrast, the strength of the evidence is high that physical activity interventions positively impact obesity prevention. Three out of three studies showed a positive impact in favor of the intervention, and all were statistically significant changes. The strength of evidence is moderate that combined diet and physical activity interventions prevent obesity or overweight in children (Table 8; Appendix F, Strength of Evidence Table 1). While 21 (81 percent) of these studies showed a favorable effect due to the intervention, only 10 (39 percent) were statistically significant. There were no studies addressing adverse events.

Intermediate Outcomes

The strength of the evidence is moderate that combined diet and physical activity interventions increase physical activity. However, the strength of the evidence is low that school/home based interventions reduce sedentary behavior, or change dietary intake (e.g., fruit and vegetable intake, energy intake, sugar-sweetened beverage intake, fatty food intake) (Appendix F, Strength of Evidence Tables 2-7).

64

Table 8. Summary of the strength of evidence for weight-related outcomes in studies taking place in a school setting with a home component

Setting	Intervention, n	Years of Publication	Enrolled Participants	Studies With Low/Moderate/High Risk of Bias(n)	% With Favorable (Statistically Sig) Outcome	% With Favorable Outcome (Does Not Need to be Stat Sig)	Risk of Bias	Consistency	Precision	Directness	Strength of the Evidence
School-Home	D, 1	1986	1,321	0/1/0	100	100	Moderate	NA	Precise	Direct	Insufficient
	PA, 3	1999-2010	1,654	1/2/0	100	100	Moderate	Consistent	Precise	Direct	High
	C, 26	1991-2012	25,438	2/20/4	39	81	Moderate	Consistent	Precise	Direct	Moderate

D = diet intervention; PA = physical activity intervention; C = combination of diet and physical activity interventions

Figure 5. Meta-analysis of change in BMI between the control group and combined diet and physical activity-only interventions in a school setting with a home component

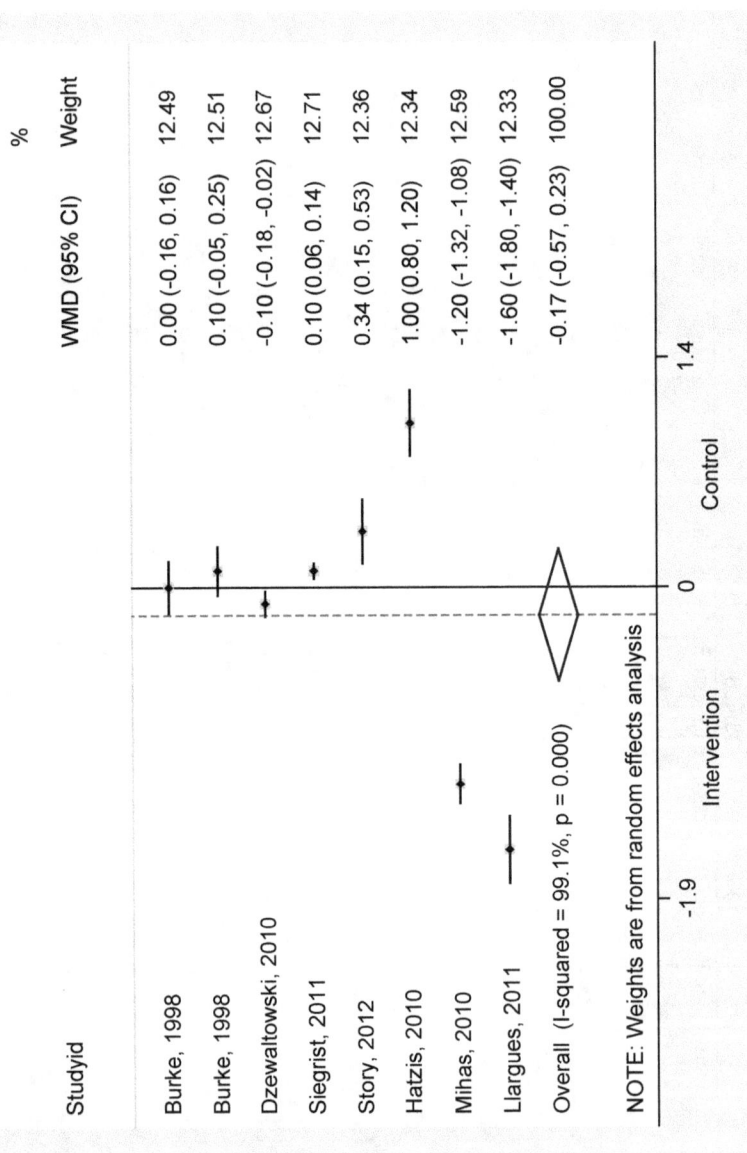

Studyid	WMD (95% CI)	% Weight
Burke, 1998	0.00 (-0.16, 0.16)	12.49
Burke, 1998	0.10 (-0.05, 0.25)	12.51
Dzewaltowski, 2010	-0.10 (-0.18, -0.02)	12.67
Siegrist, 2011	0.10 (0.06, 0.14)	12.71
Story, 2012	0.34 (0.15, 0.53)	12.36
Hatzis, 2010	1.00 (0.80, 1.20)	12.34
Mihas, 2010	-1.20 (-1.32, -1.08)	12.59
Llargues, 2011	-1.60 (-1.80, -1.40)	12.33
Overall (I-squared = 99.1%, p = 0.000)	-0.17 (-0.57, 0.23)	100.00

NOTE: Weights are from random effects analysis

WMD = weighted mean difference

School-Home-Community–Based Studies

Study Characteristics

Out of nine studies, we identified four RCTs[146-149] and five non-RCTs for this section.[150-154] Those nine studies came from 10 articles, since researchers re-analyzed results from one study[151] 4 years later using multi-level analysis and reported the findings in the most recent reference.[155] In six studies, the stated goal of the intervention was obesity prevention or weight maintenance,[147,151-154,156] while the remainder did not state a goal for the interventions.[146,148,150] One study took place in the U.S.,[147] two in the Netherlands,[148,150] two in Australia,[151,152] one in Greece,[146] one in Belgium,[149] one in Canada,[154] and the other in both Germany and Netherlands.[153] Three studies did not specify inclusion criteria,[146,151,153] while four set grade level as an inclusion criterion: two studies enrolled children from elementary and middle schools (grades 3 to 8).[148,150] The former study required schools to have (1) a certified physical education teacher, (2) a majority of pupils with low socio-economic status, and (3) a gymnasium in the school or in the immediate vicinity.[150] The latter study required participants to be able to comprehend the questionnaires and perform the fitness tests.[147] One study enrolled 4 to 12 graders.[154] Another study enrolled children from secondary school,[152] while the last one included only children from pre-elementary school to first grade.[149] Four studies also used age as an inclusion criteria, with two studies enrolling both young children and pre-adolescents (4-12 years old),[148,151] one study enrolling only adolescents (12-18 years old),[152] and one enrolled only young children (3-6 years old) (Table 9; Appendix E, Evidence Table 13).[149]

Population Characteristics

The nine studies included 14,354 participants. The percentage of girls ranged from 48 to 55.7 percent across studies. The average age of the children was under 15 years in all studies. Seven studies did not report the grade level of children,[147,149-154] one study included only children in grade 5,[146] and the remaining study's enrollment was 53 percent elementary school (grades 3-5) and 47 percent from middle school (grades 6-8).[148] Six studies did not report on race or ethnicity.[146,149,151-154] Among those that reported on race or ethnicity, one U.S.-based study included roughly 40 percent non-Hispanic white and 60 percent non-Hispanic black students.[147] The other two Dutch studies were also mixed-race studies, with one including roughly 15 percent Dutch; 31 percent Moroccan; and 55 percent Turkish, Surinam, and children of other races.[150] The other one had a large proportion of Moroccan and Turkish participants (Table 9; Appendix E, Evidence Table 14).[148]

Interventions

All the nine studies include a home and community component like involving parents and the neighboring community in the prevention programs. No studies reported on diet interventions alone. Only one study reported on a physical activity intervention alone, and this had both an educational and physical/environmental component.[150] Eight studies reported having both changes in diet and physical activity and/or other components,[146-149,151-154] with two using an educational component for diet and an educational and physical/environmental component for physical activity,[151,153] three studies using an educational and physical/environmental component for both diet and physical activity,[146,148,152] two using an educational and physical/environmental component for diet and a physical/environmental component for physical activity[147,149], and the other one using an educational component for diet and a physical/environmental component for physical activity (Table 10; Appendix E, Evidence Table 15).[154]

Table 9. Study and participant characteristics of studies based in schools with home and community components

Author, Year	RCT	Goal: Obesity Prevention	Country	Sex*	Age Range, Years*	Grade*	Other*	Total N	Followup in Weeks	% Girls†	Mean Age [Range] Years†	Grade†	Race†
Angelopoulos, 2009[146]	Y	N	Greece	NR	NR	NR	NR	646	65-73	55.7	10.3	5	NR
De Coen, 2012[149]	Y	Y	Belgium	NR	3-6	Pre-primary-1	NR	3,241	104	50	NR	NR	NR
de Meij, 2010[150]	N	N	Netherlands	NR	NR	3-8	NR	2,829	34-86	49.6	8.5	NR	Mixed, Dutch, Moroccan, Turkish, Surinam
Greening, 2011[147]	Y	Y	U.S.	NR	NR	NR	NR	450	34	48	8.3	NR	WNH, 40 % BNH, 60%
Jansen, 2011[148]	Y	N	Netherlands	NR	6-12	3-8	NR	2,622	39	Grades 3-5, 50 Grades 6-8, 50	Grades 3-5, 7.7 Grades 6-8, 10.8	Grades 3-5, Arm 1: 52.7, Arm 2: 53; Grades 6-8, Arm 1: 47.3, Arm 2: 47	Mixed, Dutch, Moroccan, Turkish, Surinam
Millar, 2011[152]	N	Y	Australia	NR	12-18	Secondary school	NR	2,054	NR	46.5	14.6 (1.42)	NR	NR
Naul, 2012[153]	N	Y	Germany, Netherlands	NR	NR	NR	NR	557	208	NR	NR	NR	NR
Sanigorski, 2008[151]	N	Y	Australia	NR	4-12	NR	NR	1,807	104-156	51	8.3	NR	NR
Tomlin, 2012[154]	N	Y	Canada	NR	NR	4-12	NR	148	28	NR	NR	NR	NR

AIAN = American Indian/Alaska Native API = Asian Pacific Islander; BMI = Body Mass Index (in kg/m^2); BNH = Black Non-Hispanic; BP = Blood Pressure; CVD = Cardio Vascular Disease;, Maint = Maintenance. Meds = Medications; N = No; NR = Not Reported; physical activity = Physical Activity; RCT = Randomized Controlled Trials; WNH = White Non-Hispanic; Y = Yes

*Inclusion/exclusion criteria

†Participant characteristics

Note: Weight outcomes were reported based on Johnson, 2012[155] for Sanigorski, 2008.[151]

Table 10. Interventions of studies based in schools with home and community components

Author, Year	Control Arm	Description of Intervention	Diet (Phys/Env)	Diet (Psych)	Physical Activity (Phys/Env)	Physical Activity (Psych)
Angelopoulos, 2009[146]	Usual care	A student workbook and teacher manual which covered themes related to self-esteem, body image, nutrition, physical activity, fitness and environmental issues.	X	X	X	X
De Coen, 2012[149]	Usual care	Intervention based on the socio-ecological model in health promotion programs. Multi-topic intervention specifically based on 'Nutrition and physical Activity Health Targets' of the Flemish Community.	X	X		X
de Meij, 2010[150]	Usual care	Offering recurrent breaks for PA, relaxation and posture exercises, during regular lessons; structural and easily accessible school sports activities. Parental information services.			X	X
Greening, 2011[147]	Usual care	Family and school-based informational events that alternated between nutrition and physical activities/contest. Health curriculum and intervention program	X	X		X
Jansen, 2011[148]	Usual care	Targets individual behaviors as well as school policies and curriculum. Parent Involvement. Local sports clubs were involved in providing some of the PE classes and PA activities outside of school hours.	X		X	X
Millar, 2011[152]	Usual care	It's Your Move Project: Use of social marketing to promote healthy eating, offering refillable water bottles at school and removing soda machines, labeled school food based on healthiness, provided recipe books . Promoted active transport to and from school, increased participation in organized sports or other recreation, and provided education sessions regarding sports. acceptance of healthy body size and shape	X	X	X	X
Naul, 2012[153]	Usual care	Multi-component program involving physical activity, nutritional lessons, etc. Home involvement of family, parents, and home life	X		X	X
Sanigorski, 2008[151]	Usual care	Community capacity-building program promoting healthy eating, physical activity and healthy weight	X	X	X	X
Tomlin, 2012[154]	baseline	Lessons on healthy eating and physical activity as well as extra physical activity sessions Promote family events	X			X

Psych = psychosocial intervention; Phys/Env = Physical/environmental intervention

70

Outcomes

Diet Interventions
None reported.

Physical Activity Interventions
One study used a physical activity intervention.[150]

Weight-Related Outcomes

BMI
The study found an nonsignificant difference between the intervention and control in BMI in favor of the control (beta=0.07 kg/m^2, 95% CI: −0.02 to 0.16 kg/m^2) (Appendix E, Evidence Table 16a).[150]

Waist Circumference
The study found a statistically nonsignificant difference between the intervention and control in waist circumference in favor of the control (beta=0.3 cm, 95% CI: −0.15 to 0.75 cm) (Appendix E, Evidence Table 16a).[150]

Clinical Outcomes
None reported.

Adverse Events
None reported.

Intermediate Outcomes
The study[150] found a significant difference between the intervention and control in organized sports participation (OR=2.8, 95% CI 2.18 to 3.62) and positive but nonsignificant improvements for physical activity (beta=40 counts/min, 95% CI −27 to 106 counts/min) and shuttle run (beta=0.02 laps, 95% CI −0.26 to 0.29 laps) (Appendix E, Evidence Table 16b).

Interpretation
We can make no conclusions. One study reported a nonsignificant change in BMI in favor of the control.[150] Based on the evidence, physical activity interventions did not significantly change weight outcomes over a period of 2 school years, as this study did not specifically target weight gain prevention but rather sports participation and aerobic fitness (which have improved significantly), thus it did not attempt to modify other risk factors for childhood obesity, such as energy intake.

Diet and Physical Activity Interventions
We identified eight studies on diet and physical activity interventions.[146-149,151-154] Six of them reported on BMI and BMI z-score,[148,149,151-154] among these two studies showed significant desirable effect.[151,152]

Weight-Related Outcomes

BMI z-Score

Five studies reported on BMI z-score.[146,149,151,152,154] Two of them found a statistically significant difference between the intervention and control in BMI z-scores (p=0.04 or 0.03),[151,152] while the other three found an nonsignificant difference between the intervention and control groups in favor of the intervention[146,149,154] (Appendix E, Evidence Table 17a,b).

BMI

Six studies reported on BMI.[146-148,151-153] Two studies found a significant difference between the intervention and control and were in favor of the intervention (p=0.03 or 0.06),[151,152] while another one with a pre-post study design reported a significant rise in BMI in followup measures as compared to baseline (p<0.001).[153] One reported by subgroups and found a positive but nonsignificant improvement in BMI for grades 3-5 (mean difference=0.10 kg/m2, 95% CI: -0.22 – 0.03 kg/m2), and almost no improvements for grades 6-8 (mean difference=0.03 kg/m2, 95% CI: -0.12-0.17 kg/m2)[148] Another two studies found a positive but nonsignificant difference between the intervention and control in BMI (Appendix E, Evidence Table 17a,b).[147,151]

BMI Percentiles

One study reported on BMI percentiles and found a desirable but nonsignificant effect (Appendix E, Evidence Table 17a, b).[147]

Prevalence of Obesity or Overweight

Two studies reported on the prevalence of obesity or overweight.[148,152] One study found a significant desirable difference between the intervention and control in the prevalence of overweight for grades 3-5 (OR=0.53, 95% CI: 0.36-0.78), but no improvements for grades 6-8 (OR=1.25, 95% CI: 0.79-1.99).[148] The other one found an expected but nonsignificant difference between the intervention and control in the prevalence of obesity or overweight (p=0.12) (Appendix E, Evidence Table 17a,b).[152]

Percent Body Fat

Two studies reported on body fat percentage. One found a significant difference between the intervention and control in body fat percentage in favor of the intervention (p=0.02),[147] and the other found a favorable but nonsignificant intervention effect (p=0.58)[152] (Appendix E, Evidence Table 17a,b).

Waist Circumference

Three studies reported on waist circumference.[147,148,151] One study reported by subgroups and found a significant difference between the intervention and control for grades 3-5 in favor of the intervention (difference in mean change=-1.29 cm, 95% CI: -2.16 – -0.42 cm), as well as an expected although nonsignificant difference between the intervention and control for grades 6-8 (difference in mean change=-0.71cm, 95% CI: -1.72 – 0.29 cm).[148] One study[147] found a favorable but nonsignificant difference between the intervention and control (p=0.92). The other study found a statistically significant difference between the intervention and control in favor of the intervention (p<0.05) (Appendix E, Evidence Table 17a,b).[151]

Weight

Three studies reported on body weight.[151,152,157] Two studies[151,152] found a significant desirable intervention effect (p=0.03 or 0.04), while the other found a favorable but nonsignificant difference between the intervention and control groups (p=0.124)[146] (Appendix E, Evidence Table 17a,b).

Weight/Height Ratio

One study reported weight/height ratio and found a significant intervention effect (p=0.01) (Appendix E, Evidence Table 17a, b).[151]

Clinical Outcomes

Two studies reported on change in clinical outcomes.[146,154] One study found a significant difference between the intervention and control in systolic and diastolic blood pressures in favor of the intervention (p=0.016 for systolic and p=0.005 for diastolic blood pressure).[146] The other study with a pre-post study design found an increase in systolic blood pressure z-scores (p=0.076) and a decrease in diastolic blood pressure z-scores (p=0.267), but both were nonsignificant (Appendix E, Evidence Table 17c).[154]

Adverse Events

A single study reported on potential adverse events.[151] The study examined a number of safety measures and concluded that the intervention did not increase the proportion of children participating in behaviors that would put them at increased risk of eating disorders (p-value not reported). Specifically, the intervention did not increase the prevalence of thinness/underweight (intervention: 3.1 percent at baseline to 3.6 percent at followup, comparison: 2.2–2.4 percent, not significant) (Appendix E, Evidence Table 17d).[151]

Intermediate Outcomes

Physical Activity and Sedentary Behavior

Seven studies reported on changes in physical activity.[149-152,154] Two studies reported on a combination of diet, physical activity, and self-management and found a significant desirable effect on physical activity levels (p=0.04 or 0.041).[146,147]

Three studies reported on a combination of diet and physical activity and found an undesirable intervention effect; one study was statistically significant (p=0.01)[152] and the other two were not (p=0.555 or not reported).[149,154] Two studies reported a favorable but nonsignificant intervention effect (p-value not reported).[150,151]

Three studies reported on a combination of diet and physical activity reported on changes in sedentary behavior.[149,151,152] One study found an unexpected but significant intervention effect (p=0.001),[152] one found a desirable intervention effect with unknown significance,[151] while the other one found no difference in change in sedentary behavior between the intervention and control groups (Appendix E, Evidence Table 17e).[149]

Dietary Intake

We identified nine studies that examined dietary intake. One study reported on change in calorie intake, which showed no significant desirable effect. Five studies reported on change in fruit and vegetable intake. One of these, which intervened on a combination of diet, physical activity and self-management, showed significant desirable effect. Three studies reported on change in fatty food intake. Of these, two that intervened on a combination of diet, physical activity and self-management showed significant desirable effect. Five studies reported on change in sugar-sweetened beverage intake, and one of them showed significant desirable effect, which intervened on a combination of diet, physical activity and self-management. Seven studies reported on change in physical activity levels, and two of them showed significant desirable effect, which both intervened on a combination of diet, physical activity and self-management. Three studies reported on change in sugar-sweetened beverage intake, and none showed significant desirable effect.

Only one study, examining a combination of diet and physical activity, reported on change in calorie intake and found a nonsignificant difference in calorie intake between the intervention and control in favor of the intervention (p=0.159).[154]

Five studies reported on change in fruit and vegetable intake.[146,149,151,152,154] Four studies found a favorable intervention effect,[146,149,151,154] however, in three of the studies examining a combination of diet and physical activity, the findings were either nonsignificant or the studies did not report on significance.[149,151,154] Only one study, examining a combination of diet, physical activity, and self-management, showed significant desirable effect (p=0.044).[146] The last study reported on a combination of diet and physical activity and found an undesirable intervention effect in fruit and vegetable intake (p=0.14).[152]

Three studies reported on change in fatty foods intake. Two studies reported on a combination of diet, physical activity, and self-management and found a significant desirable effect (p=0.0005 or 0.028).[146,147] The other study reported on a combination of diet and physical activity and found an nonsignificant difference in fatty foods intake between the intervention and control in favor of the intervention (p=0.054).[154]

Five studies reported on change in sugar-sweetened beverage intake.[146,149,151,152,154] One study reported on a combination of diet, physical activity, and self-management and found a significant desirable effect on sugar-sweetened beverage intake (p=0.039).[146] Three studies reported on a combination of diet and physical activity and found an undesirable intervention effect,[149,152,154] while the other study reported on a combination of diet and physical activity and found a favorable intervention effect in sugar-sweetened beverage intake,[151] however, it did not report the p-value.

Interpretation

The results from an outcome measure from each of the eight studies reporting on combined diet and physical activity interventions support our conclusions. Five studies reported on BMI z-score.[146,149,151,152,154] All reported changes in BMI z-score in favor of the intervention. Two studies were significant,[151,152] and the remaining three reported an nonsignificant change.[146,149,154] Three studies reported on BMI.[147,148,153] One reported an nonsignificant change in BMI in favor of the intervention.[147] One reported an nonsignificant change in BMI in favor of the intervention for grades 3-5, but almost no improvements for grades 6-8[148]. Another pre-post study found a significant rise in BMI in followup measures as compared to baseline disfavor of the intervention.[153] Based on this evidence, we conclude that studies on combined diet and physical activity interventions in a school, home, and community setting generally showed positive but nonsignificant improvements in weight outcomes over a period of at least 6 months because the majority of these studies specifically targeted weight gain prevention; all included both dietary and physical activity components focusing both on education and making structural changes to promote diet and physical activity. One reason for the nonsignificant effect of some of the interventions on weight outcomes might be that that the interventions did not specifically target weight gain prevention, or the sample size was too small to detect a significant effect.

Strength of the Evidence

Weight-Related Outcomes

The strength of evidence is insufficient that school-home-community based interventions that only attempt to change physical activity can prevent obesity or overweight in children, as there was only one study with moderate risk of bias. The strength of evidence is high that interventions which use a combination of interventions (e.g., diet, physical activity, and/or self-management) can prevent obesity or overweight in children, as both a study with low risk of bias and the majority of studies with moderate risk of bias showed a favorable effect (Table 11; Appendix F, Strength of Evidence Table 1).

Intermediate Outcomes

There was insufficient evidence to grade calorie or fatty foods intake in interventions that included a combination of diet and physical activity approaches in a school-home-community setting, as there was only one study with moderate risk of bias. The strength of evidence is low to grade changes in sugar-sweetened beverage intake, physical activity levels, or sedentary behaviors for interventions trying to impact both diet and physical activity, as there were a few studies with low or moderate risk of bias and they showed conflicting results. The strength of evidence is moderate that diet and physical activity approaches impact fruit and vegetable intake in a school-home-community setting, as both a study with low risk of bias and another study with moderate risk of bias showed a favorable effect (and there were no low or moderate risk of bias studies going in the other direction).

The strength of evidence is insufficient that interventions which included diet, physical activity, and self-management impact fruit and vegetable intake or sugar-sweetened beverage intake in a school-home-community setting, as there was only one study with moderate risk of bias in this category. The strength of evidence is moderate that interventions which included diet, physical activity, and self-management impact fatty foods intake or physical activity levels in a school-home-community setting, as there were only two studies with a moderate risk of bias that both reported a favorable intervention effect (Appendix F, Strength of Evidence Tables 2-7).

Table 11. Summary of the strength of evidence for weight-related outcomes in studies taking place in schools with a home and community component

Setting	Intervention, n	Years of Publication	Enrolled Participants	Studies With Low/ Moderate/ High Risk of Bias(n)	% With Favorable (Statistically Sig) Outcome	% With Favorable Outcome (Does Not Need to be Stat Sig)	Risk of Bias	Consistency	Precision	Directness	Strength of the Evidence
School-	PA, 1	2010	2,829	0/1/0	0	0	Moderate	NA	Precise	Direct	Insufficient
Home- Community	C, 8	2008-2012	11,525	1/4/3	12.5	81	Moderate	Consistent	Imprecise	Direct	High

School-Community–Based Studies

Study Characteristics

We included six school/community-based studies including three RCTs[158-160] and three non-RCTs (Table 12; Appendix E, Evidence Table 18).[161-163] The stated goal in four studies was obesity prevention or weight maintenance.[158,160,161,163] Three studies took place in the U.S.,[159,160,162] one in Germany,[158] one in Canada,[161] and the other one in New Zealand.[163] Two studies did not list any inclusion criteria.[161,162] One included only English-speaking girls from one public middle school (grade 6).[159] One included kindergarten to Grade 2 Latinos.[160] One included only children aged 9 to 13 years.[163] The other study included children (grades 2 to 3) from elementary schools in socially deprived neighborhoods of two cities in Germany (Table 12; Appendix E, Evidence Table 18).[158]

Population Characteristics

The six studies enrolled 10,087 children. Two studies did not report the distribution of gender,[160,161] one included only girls,[159] and the other three studies included 48.0 to 51.6 percent girls.[158,162,163] Two studies did not report age,[160,163] one study did not report age but included only children from grade 6,[159] the remaining three studies enrolled children from elementary school.[158,161,162] Only one study reported on race or ethnicity, and included 46 percent white children, 24 percent black children, 12 percent Hispanic children, and 18 percent children of other races or with unknown race,[159] another two studies also included a sample of mixed races/ethnicities (Table 12; Appendix E, Evidence Table 19).[162,163]

Interventions

Out of six studies, one reported on diet, one on physical activity, and the remaining four reported on a combination of diet and physical activity. One study reported on a diet intervention[158] that included both educational and physical/environmental components to alter diet. Two studies reported on both diet and physical activity components and used both an educational and physical/environmental approach.[161,163] One intervention attempted to modify diet from both a psychosocial and physical/environmental approach, and attempted to modify physical activity from a psychosocial approach.[162] Another study included three active arms, with each arm attempting to modify both diet and physical activity: one used a psychosocial approach, another used a physical/environmental approach, and the final arm used both approaches.[160] Another study included physical activity (both educational and physical/environmental) interventions and self-management (Table 13; Appendix E, Evidence Table 20).[159]

77

Table 12. Study and participant characteristics of studies based in schools with a community component

Author, Year	RCT	Goal: Obesity Prevention	Country	Sex*	Age Range, Years*	Grade*	Other*	Total N	Followup in Weeks	% Girls[†]	Mean Age [Range] Years[†]	Grade[†]	Race[†]
Crespo, 2012[160]	Y	Y	U.S.	NR	NR	K-2	Latino	820	156	NR	NR	NR	NR
Macaulay, 1997[161]	N	Y	Canada	NR	NR	NR	NR	537	156	NR	[6-11]	1-6	NR
Madsen, 2009[162]	N	N	U.S.	NR	NR	NR	NR	178	34	48	9.8 (7.9-12.2)	3-5	Mixed, White, Black, Latino/Hispanic, Asian/Pacific Islander, Other/unknown
Muckelbauer, 2009[158]	Y	Y	Germany	NR	NR	2-3	NR	2,950	47	49.8	Arm 1: 8.3 Arm 2: 8.3	2-3	NR
Utter, 2011[163]	N	Y	New Zealand	NR	9-13	NR	NR	3,881	104	51.6	NR	NR	Mixed, Asian/Pacific Islander, Pacific, Maori, European
Webber, 2008[159]	Y	NR	U.S.	Girls	NR	6	NR	1,721	156	100	NR	6	WNH: 46.1%; BNH: 23.5%; Latino/Hispanic: 12.3%; Multi-ethnic, or missing: 18.0%

BNH = Black non-Hispanic; N = no; NR = not reported; RCT = randomized controlled trials; WNH=White non-Hispanic; Y = yes

*Inclusion/exclusion criteria.

[†]Participant characteristics.

Table 13. Interventions of studies based in schools with a community component

Author, Year	Control Arm	Description of Intervention	Diet (Phys/Env)	Diet (Psych)	Physical Activity (Phys/Env)	Physical Activity (Psych)
Crespo, 2012[160]	Usual care	Intervention delivered by a community health advisor through home visit focused on increasing fruit, vegetable, and water consumption, increasing active play and decreasing sugar-sweetened beverages and TV viewing	X		X	
	Usual care	Implementation and improvement of cafeteria salad bars. School playground improvement Improvement of community park Health Informatics:		X		X
	Usual care	Intervention delivered by a community health advisor through home visit focused on increasing fruit, vegetable, and water consumption. School playground improvement . Improvement of community park.	X	X	X	X
Macaulay, 1997[161]	Usual care	Storytelling, games, food tasting, experiments, puppet shows, crafts, and audiovisual presentations to promote healthy eating. Emphasizes the benefits and pleasure of daily physical activity and the different types of activity: aerobic, strength building, and flexibility	X		X	
Madsen, 2009[162]	Usual care	Play soccer three days a week Literacy improvement: participants perform community service or undertake creative writing the remaining two days a week.			X	
Muckelbauer, 2009[158]	Usual care	Combined environmental and educational intervention solely promoting water consumption	X	X		

Psych = psychosocial intervention; Phys/Env = Physical/environmental intervention

Outcomes

Diet Intervention

Two articles (representing one study) investigated the impact of diet interventions on childhood obesity prevention.[158,164]

Weight-Related Outcomes

BMI

The study significantly lowered BMI in the intervention group versus in the control group after intervention (p=0.037). There was no significant difference before intervention (Appendix E, Evidence Table 21a).[158]

Prevalence of Obesity or Overweight

A primary study found significant improvements in the intervention group versus in the control group, as the incidence rate for obesity was significantly lower in the intervention group (p=0.018). The remission rate (previously overweight or obese to normal weight) for obesity or overweight was also higher in the intervention group but did not reach statistical significance (p=0.485 or 0.251) (Appendix E, Evidence Table 21a).[158]

Stratified results in another study, based on immigration backgrounds,[164] found significant improvements in the incidence of overweight (p=0.006) and positive but nonsignificant improvements in the remission rate (p=0.11) in the non-immigrant group immigrants; and positive but nonsignificant improvements in the incidence rate of overweight (p=0.99) and no improvements in the remission rate (p=0.23) in the immigrant group.

Clinical Outcomes

None reported.

Adverse Events

None reported.

Intermediate Outcomes

Dietary Intake

The study found significant improvements in water and soft drinks/juices consumption post intervention (p<0.001 and p=0.019) in the intervention but not in the control (p= 0.576 and p = 0.670).[158]

Another study reported on immigrant and non-immigrant subgroups.[164] Water consumption had improved significantly in both subgroups, with positive but nonsignificant improvements in juice consumption and no improvements in soft drinks consumption in both subgroups (Appendix E, Evidence Table 21b).

Interpretation

The results of the outcomes measures in one study reporting the effect of diet intervention on BMI and prevalence of overweight and obesity support our conclusions. The one study reported on a statistically significant change in BMI in favor of the intervention.[158] Based on the evidence, we conclude that this diet intervention showed significant improvements in BMI and prevalence of overweight and obesity over a period of 47 weeks because it specifically targeted weight gain prevention and the sample size was as big as 2,950.

Physical Activity Intervention

Weight-Related Outcomes

BMI
A single study reported no improvements for BMI (p-value not reported) (Appendix E, Evidence Table 22a).[159]

Percent Body Fat
One study reported no improvements for percent body fat (p-value not reported) (Appendix E, Evidence Table 22a).[159]

Skinfold Thickness
A study found positive but nonsignificant improvements for triceps skinfold thickness (p-value not reported) (Appendix E, Evidence Table 22a).[159]

Weight
This study found positive but nonsignificant improvements for body weight (p-value not reported) (Appendix E, Evidence Table 22a).[159]

Clinical Outcomes
None reported.

Adverse Events
None reported.

Intermediate Outcomes

Physical Activity and Sedentary Behavior
This study measured physical activity using multiple scales. Change in minutes of moderate to vigorous physical activity, and change in minutes of total physical activity were positive but nonsignificant. Change in sedentary behavior was also positive but nonsignificant (p-value not reported) (Appendix E, Evidence Table 22b).[159]

Interpretation
We can make no conclusions regarding the effect of a physical activity intervention on BSI. The one study reported no change in BMI.[159] Based on the evidence, this physical activity intervention among girls showed no improvements in weight outcomes over a period of 3 years because it did not specifically target weight gain prevention, and the effect may have faded over 3 years.

Diet and Physical Activity Intervention
We identified four studies.[160-163]

Weight-Related Outcomes

BMI z-Score
Three studies measured the impact of diet and physical activity interventions on BMI z-scores.[160,162,163] The intervention was effective in reducing BMI z-scores in two studies but both were nonsignificant,[160,162] another pre-post study reported nonsignificant increase in followup compared to baseline (p=0.13) (Appendix E, Evidence Table 23a,b).[163]

BMI
Three studies in this setting measured the impact of diet and physical activity interventions on BMI.[161-163] The intervention was effective in reducing BMI in two studies,[161,162] with one reporting significant improvements (p<0.01).[161] Another pre-post study reported nonsignificant increase in followup compared to baseline (p=0.18) (Appendix E, Evidence Table 23a,b).[163]

Prevalence of Overweight and Obesity
Once study reported on prevalence of obesity and found that it declined from 33 percent at baseline to 27 percent at followup (p = 0.103) (Appendix E, Evidence Table 23a,b).[162]

Percent Body Fat
Once study reported on percent body fat and found a nonsignificant difference between the intervention and control in favor of the control (p = 0.16) (Appendix E, Evidence Table 23a,b).[163]

Skinfold Thickness
One study reported on triceps skinfold thickness and sub-scapular skinfold thickness and found a significant desirable effect in favor of the intervention (p-value not reported) (Appendix E, Evidence Table 23a,b).[161]

Weight
One study reported on weight and found a nonsignificant difference between the intervention and control in favor of the control (p = 0.21) (Appendix E, Evidence Table 23a,b).[163]

Clinical Outcomes
None reported.

Adverse Events
None reported.

Intermediate Outcomes

Physical Activity and Sedentary Behavior
Two studies reported on changes in physical activity levels, with one reporting a desirable but nonsignificant intervention effect (p=0.61),[160] and the other finding no effect (p=0.65).[163] Two studies reported on sedentary behavior, both found a desirable but nonsignificant effect (p=0.58 and p=0.09) (Appendix E, Evidence Table 23c).[160,163]

Dietary Intake

One study reported on changes in fruit and vegetable intake and showed a favorable but nonsignificant intervention effect (p=0.75).[160] One study reported on changes in sugar-sweetened beverage intake and found a favorable but nonsignificant effect (p=0.42) (Appendix E, Evidence Table 23c).[163]

Interpretation

The results from an outcome measure from each of the four studies support that combined diet physical activity interventions generally showed positive but nonsignificant improvements in weight outcomes over a period of at least 6 months because the sample size was usually too small (e.g. 178 participants in one study).. Three studies reported on BMI z-scores.[160,162,163] Two studies reported changes in BMI z-score in favor of the intervention and both were nonsignificant.[160,162] One pre-post study reported changes in BMI z-score from baseline to followup disfavor of the intervention.[163] One study reported on BMI and reported a significant change in favor of the intervention.[161]

Strength of the Evidence

Weight-Related Outcomes

The strength of evidence is insufficient that a solely diet or physical activity approach can impact weight outcomes in a school and community setting as only one study addressed each. The strength of evidence is moderate that combined diet and physical activity approaches prevent overweight or obesity in a school and community setting, as the two studies with moderate risk of bias showed a favorable effect and there was no other low risk of bias studies in the opposite direction. Three of these four studies showed a desirable intervention effect, while only one of them was statistically significant (Table 14; Appendix F, Strength of Evidence Table 1).

Intermediate Outcomes

The strength of evidence is insufficient that diet and physical activity approaches impact fruit and vegetable intake or sugar-sweetened beverage intake in a community/school-based setting as there was only one study in this category. The strength of evidence is low that diet and physical activity approaches impact physical activity or sedentary behaviors in a community/school-based setting as there was only one study with moderate risk of bias that reported a favorable effect and the other one was a study with high risk of bias. The strength of evidence is low that interventions which included physical activity and self-management impact BMI in a community/school-based setting as there were only two studies with high risk of bias that reported a desirable effect (Appendix F, Strength of Evidence Tables 4-7).

Table 14. Summary of the strength of evidence for weight-related outcomes in studies taking place in schools with a community component

Setting	Intervention, n	Years of Publication	Enrolled Participants	Studies with Low/ Moderate/ High Risk of Bias(n)	% With Favorable (Statistically Sig) Outcome	% With Favorable Outcome (Does Not Need to be Stat Sig)	Risk of Bias	Consistency	Precision	Directness	Strength of the Evidence
School- Community	D, 1	2009	2,950	0/1/0	100	100	Moderate	NA	Precise	Direct	Insufficient
	PA, 1	2008	1,721	0/0/1	0	0	High	NA	Imprecise	Direct	Insufficient
	C, 4	1997-2012	3,017	0/2/2	25	75	Moderate	Consistent	Imprecise	Direct	Moderate

D = diet intervention; PA = physical activity intervention; C = combination of diet and physical activity interventions

84

School-Consumer Health Informatics–Based Studies

Study Characteristics

We included four studies.[165-168] One study used a quasi-experimental design[165] and the other studies were RCTs.[166-168] Two of the studies stated weight maintenance as the goal of the interventions and took place in the Netherlands.[167,168] One study took place in the U.S.[166] Three of the four studies listed grade level as inclusion criteria. One study included participants in grades 4 and 5,[166] another study included participants in grades 10 and 11,[165] and a third study included participants in the first year of secondary school (Table 15, Appendix E, Evidence Table 24).[167]

Population Characteristics

The number of participants in the four included studies was 3,231 children.[165-168] In the four studies the total followup period reported for participants ranged between 26 to 114 weeks. Three studies reported mean age[165,167,168] and it ranged between 12.6 to 15.04 years. One study included only girls[165] and the percent girl participants ranged from 41.1 percent to 50.3 percent in two other studies.[167,168] All children in one study were in grades 4 and 5[166] while participants in another study were in grades 10 and 11.[165] In one study, 57 percent of participants were white, 20 percent were Latino/Hispanic, and 17 percent were Asian/Pacific Islander. In another study[167] 82.3 percent of participants were classified as Western and 17.7 percent of participants as Non-Western. In a third study reporting race, 66 to 78.9 percent of participants were Western and 21.1 to 34 percent of participants were Non-Western (Table 15, Appendix E, Evidence Table 25).[168]

Interventions

Two studies reported on physical activity interventions.[165,167] One study described an intervention consisting of supervised in-class activity, health education, and Internet-based self-monitoring components.[165] This intervention lasted 30 weeks and aimed to increase levels of physical activity. Participants received 60-minute long educational discussions once a week related to the health benefits of exercise and strategies for adopting an active lifestyle. Student input influenced activity choices, which included a variety of aerobic and strength-building activities. Participants reported physical activity via Internet-based self-monitoring. Another study[167] reported on a 3-week web-based intervention that promoted physical activity among participants. Individuals in both intervention arms received school-based online lessons focused on improving physical activity and goal setting. Additionally, participants randomized to the YouRaction+e arm received computer-assisted feedback on the availability of physical activity facilities in their residential neighborhoods (Table 16, Appendix E, and Evidence Table 26).[165,167]

Two studies reported on diet and physical activity interventions.[166,168] One study[166] randomized participants to attend the multidisciplinary Wellness, Academics and You program for 1 school year. The intervention consisted of a five-module program intended to develop their health attitudes and behavior addressing nutrition, physical activity, and self-management. The intervention group participated in a variety of activities integrated into their core curriculum. Activity duration ranged from 20 minutes to more than 1 hour. Another study[168] reported on a 10-week Web-based intervention that aimed to promote healthy diet, increase physical activity, and reduce sedentary behavior. Participants also received lessons focused on weight management, goal setting, and behavioral feedback (Table 16, Appendix E, and Evidence Table 26).[166,168]

Table 15. Study and participant characteristics of studies based in schools with a consumer health informatics component

Author, Year	RCT	Goal: Obesity Prevention	Country	Sex*	Age Range, Years*	Grade*	Other*	Total N	Followup in Weeks	% Girls[†]	Mean Age [Range] Years[†]	Grade[†]	Race[†]
Schneider, 2007[165]	N	N	NR	NR	NR	10-11		122	30	100	15.04	NR	WNH: 57% Latino/ Hispanic: 20% API: 17%
Spiegel, 2006[166]	Y	N	U.S.	NR	NR	4-5		1,013	34	NR	NR	4-5	NR
Prins, 2012[167]	Y	Y	Netherlands	NR	12-13	First year of secondary school	Attend participating school in the Rotterdam Area	1,213	26	Arm1: 46.6 Arm2: 47.2 Arm3: 49	Arm1: 12.6(0.4) Arm2: 12.7(0.5) Arm3: 12.7(0.5)	NR	Western Overall:(82.3) Arm1:(74.8) Arm2:(77.9) Non-Western (Overall:(17.7) Arm1:(25.2) Arm2:(22.1)
Ezendam, 2012[168]	Y	Y	Netherlands	NR	12-13	NR	Secondary school; Participants in 1-5 first year classes	883	114	Arm1: 50.3 Arm2: 41.1	Arm1: 12.6(0.6) Arm2: 12.7(0.7)	NR	Western Arm1:314(78.9) Arm2:320(66.0) Non-WesternArm1:84(21.1) Arm2:165(34.0)

API = Asian Pacific Islander; N = no; NR = not reported; RCT = randomized controlled trials; WNH = White non-Hispanic; Y = yes
*Inclusion/exclusion criteria.
[†]Participant characteristics.

87

Table 16. Interventions of studies based in schools with a consumer health informatics component

Author, Year	Control Arm	Description of Intervention	Diet (Phys/Env)	Diet (Psych)	Physical Activity (Phys/Env)	Physical Activity (Psych)
Ezendam, 2012[168]	Usual care	Web-based computer lessons conducted by teacher with a health informatics computer-tailored intervention	X		X	
Prins, 2012[167]	Usual care	School based online lessons Web-based computer tailored physical activity promotion intervention			X	
	Usual care	School based online lessons plus feedback on nearby physical activity facilities Web-based computer tailored PA promotion intervention			X	
Schneider, 2007[165]	Usual care	Increase students' levels of physical activity through supervised in-class activity, health education, and Internet-based self-monitoring			X	X

Psych = psychosocial intervention; Phys/Env = physical/environmental intervention

88

Outcomes

Diet Interventions
None reported.

Physical Activity Intervention
Two studies evaluated the effect of a physical activity intervention on weight outcomes.[165,167] One quasi-experimental study included only adolescent girls [165] and the other study[167] randomized adolescents to a control or one of two intervention groups.

Weight-Related Outcomes

BMI Percentile
One study reported a small increase in BMI over time in the intervention group, compared to the control group. (Appendix E, Evidence Table 27).[165]

Prevalence of Overweight and Obesity
One study reported no statistically significant difference between either intervention group and control in percent overweight or obese (Evidence Table 27).[167]

Percent Body Fat
One study reported no difference between the intervention and control in percent body fat over time. (Appendix E, Evidence Table 27)[165]

Waist Circumference
One study reported no statistically significant difference between either intervention group and control in waist circumference (Evidence Table 27).[167]

Clinical Outcomes
One study measured peak oxygen consumption and VO2 peak (L/min).[165] Peak oxygen consumption increased in the intervention group; this was a significant difference between the intervention and control ($p=0.001$). VO2 peak increased in the intervention group with a p-value of 0.02. (Appendix E, Evidence Table 27).

Adverse Events
None reported.

Intermediate Outcomes

Physical Activity and Sedentary Behavior
In one study,[167] there was no statistically significant difference between either intervention group and control in minutes of moderate-to-vigorous physical activity or compliance with moderate-to-vigorous physical activity guidelines (Evidence Table 27).[167]

Interpretation
The results from an outcome measure from each of the two studies reporting on physical activity interventions support our conclusions--none of the school with consumer health

informatics physical activity interventions showed a significant beneficial effect on weight outcomes. One study reported on BMI percentiles and reported a small nonsignificant change in favor of the intervention.[169] The other study reported no statistically significant change in prevalence of overweight or obesity.[167] Based on this evidence we cannot determine if physical activity interventions impact BMI percentiles or prevalence of overweight and obesity.

These studies may be limited by exclusion of concurrent nutrition education and short followup. Additional factors that may have limited the realization of an intervention effect in one of the studies[165] include use of a non-randomized study design.

Diet and Physical Activity Interventions

Two studies evaluated the effect of a diet and physical activity intervention on weight outcomes.[166,168] One study randomly assigned 1,013 students in grade 4 and 5 from 69 classes in four states to intervention or control groups.[166] Another study randomized 883 adolescents to an intervention or control group.[168]

Weight-Related Outcomes

BMI
In one study,[166] there was a significant difference between the intervention and control in BMI. The shift in BMI from baseline to after intervention was significant (Pearson correlation coefficient = -0.186, $p = 0.01$ level) In a second study[168], there was no intervention effect on BMI at followup (Appendix E, Evidence Table 28a,b).[166,168]

One study[168] reported no intervention effect on BMI among subgroups of overweight or obese children (Appendix E, Evidence Table 28a,b).

Prevalence of Overweight and Obesity
One study[166] reported a notable decrease in the intervention group in the prevalence of obesity, and the decrease was most significant for overweight participants. The study did not statistically analyze this difference in change of the prevalence. In a second study[168] there was no intervention effect on the prevalence (Appendix E, Evidence Table 28a,b).[166,168]

One study[168] reported no intervention effect on prevalence of overweight or obese among subgroups of overweight or obese children (Appendix E, Evidence Table 28a,b).

Waist Circumference
One study[168] reported no intervention effect on waist circumference among overweight or obese children (Appendix E, Evidence Table 28a,b).[168]

Clinical Outcome
None reported.

Adverse Events
None reported.

Intermediate Outcomes

Physical Activity and Sedentary Activity

Two studies addressed change in physical activity. One reported a change in favor of the intervention, but the change was not significant.[168] The other reported a change in favor of the control, but this change was not significant.[166] A third study reported on change in sedentary behavior by measuring changes in screen time (TV, video games). This study reported a change in favor of the intervention but reported no significance values (Appendix E, Evidence Table 28c).[168]

Dietary Intake

In one study, the combined diet and physical activity intervention compared to the control group resulted in higher fruit and vegetable consumption and increased physical activity.[166] The study did not statistically analyze this difference in change in physical activity and fruit and vegetable intake. In another study,[168] compared to the control, the intervention group had lower self-reported snack consumption, were less likely to report drinking more than 400ml of sugar-sweetened beverages per day, and reported more vegetable consumption. While these between-group differences in dietary outcomes were observed at 4-month followup, they were not sustained at the 2-year followup. In this same study there was no significant intervention effect on physical activity (Appendix E, Evidence Table 28c).[166,168]

Interpretation

The results from outcome measures from two studies reporting on combined diet and physical activity interventions support our conclusions-- we cannot determine if combined diet and physical activity interventions impact BMI. These two studies reported on BMI.[166,168] One showed a significant change in favor of the intervention,[166] and the other showed no intervention effect.[168]

Strength of the Evidence

Weight-Related Outcomes

The strength of evidence is insufficient that school with consumer health informatics physical activity interventions prevent obesity or overweight in children. We graded this body as insufficient because it lacked precision and included studies with moderate risk of bias. The strength of evidence is insufficient that combination diet and physical activity interventions prevent obesity or overweight in children. We graded this body as insufficient because it lacked precision and included studies with moderate risk of bias (Table 17, Appendix F, Strength of Evidence Table 1).

Intermediate Outcomes

The strength of evidence is insufficient that school-based physical activity interventions with consumer health informatics change physical activity. The strength of evidence is insufficient that combined diet and physical activity interventions impact changes in sedentary behavior or fruit and vegetable intake. One study each reported on these intermediate outcomes and neither presented precision (Appendix F, Strength of Evidence Tables 4-6).

The strength of the evidence that diet and physical activity interventions impact change in physical activity and change in fruit and vegetable intake is insufficient. Two moderate risk of bias studies with inconsistent results reported on these outcomes and did not report precision (Appendix F).

Table 17. Summary of the strength of evidence for weight-related outcomes in studies taking place in a school setting with a consumer health informatics component

Setting	Intervention, n	Years of Publication	Enrolled Participants	Studies With Low/Moderate/High Risk of Bias(n)	% With Favorable (Statistically Sig) Outcome	% With Favorable Outcome (Does Not Need to be Stat Sig)	Risk of Bias	Consistency	Precision	Directness	Strength of the Evidence
School-CHI	PA,2	2007-2012	1,335	0/2/0	0	0	Moderate	Inconsistent	Imprecise	Direct	Insufficient
	C, 2	2006-2012	1,896	0/2/0	50	50	Moderate	Inconsistent	Imprecise	Direct	Insufficient

PA = physical activity intervention; C = combination of diet and physical activity interventions; CHI = consumer health informatics; sig = significant

School-Home-Consumer Health Informatics–Based Studies

Study Characteristics

We included only one non-RCT.[170] The goal of the intervention in this study was weight maintenance and the study took place in England. Primary schools were the only inclusion criteria (Table 18; Evidence Table 24).[170]

Population Characteristics

One study included 589 participants followed them over a period of 120 weeks.[170] The mean age for the control group was 8.86 years and for the control group 8.76 years. The study enrolled 94.8 to 96.5 percent white participants and did not report the percentage of girls or the grade level (Table 18; Evidence Table 25).[170]

Interventions

One study reported on a 40-week diet and physical activity intervention.[170] This intervention promoted physical activity through the provision of physical education lessons, and target activities (1 mile run/walk). Additionally, participants received CD-rom based learning exercises on healthy eating and physical activity and along with their families were able to access an interactive website reinforcing key messages of the intervention (Table 19; Evidence Table 26).[170]

Table 18. Study and participant characteristics of studies based in schools with a home and consumer health informatics component

Author, Year	RCT	Goal: Obesity Prevention	Country	Sex*	Age Range, Years*	Grade*	Other*	Total N	Followup in Weeks	% Girls[†]	Mean Age [Range] Years[†]	Grade[†]	Race[†]
Gorely, 2011[170]	N	Y	England	NR	NR		Primary School	589	120	NR	Arm 1: 8.86 Arm 2: 8.76	NR	NR

N = no; NR = not reported; RCT = randomized controlled trials; Y = yes
*inclusion/exclusion criteria.
[†]participant characteristics.

Table 19. Interventions of studies based in schools with a home and consumer health informatics component

Author, Year	Control Arm	Description of Intervention	Diet (Phys/Env)	Diet (Psych)	Physical Activity (Phys/Env)	Physical Activity (Psych)
Gorely, 2011[170]	Usual care	GreatFun2Run: Classroom and physical education sessions Interactive website for parents and children Local media campaign to promote healthy nutrition and Physical activity.	X		X	X

Psych = psychosocial intervention; Phys/Env = physical/environmental intervention

95

Outcomes

Diet Interventions
None reported.

Physical Activity Interventions
None reported.

Diet and Physical Activity Interventions
One study evaluated the effect of a diet and physical activity intervention on weight outcomes.[170] The study non-randomly assigned 589 students to an intervention or matched control group.[170]

Weight-Related Outcomes

BMI
There was no significant difference in BMI between the intervention and control groups (Appendix F, Evidence Table 28a).[170]

Percent Body Fat
Among participants in the intervention group, there was a significant increase in percent body fat compared to the control (Appendix F, Evidence Table 28a,b).[170]

Waist Circumference
There was no significant difference in BMI between the intervention and control groups (Appendix F, Evidence Table 28a,b).[170]

Clinical Outcome
None reported.

Adverse Events
None reported.

Intermediate Outcome
There was no significant difference between the intervention group and control in minutes per day of moderate-to-vigorous physical activity (Appendix F, Evidence Table 28c).[170]

Interpretation
We can make no conclusions. This study showed no intervention effect of combined diet and physical activity.[170] Based on this evidence we cannot determine if combined diet physical activity interventions impact BMI.

Strength of the Evidence

Weight-Related Outcomes

The strength of evidence is insufficient that school, home, consumer health informatics diet and physical activity interventions prevent obesity or overweight in children. We graded this body as insufficient because it included only a single study with high risk of bias. No studies measured adverse events (Table 20, Appendix F, Strength of Evidence Table 1).

Intermediate Outcomes

The strength of the evidence is insufficient that combined diet and physical activity interventions impact change in physical activity. A single high risk of bias study was not sufficient enough evidence to draw a conclusion (Appendix F, Strength of Evidence Table 6).

Table 20. Summary of the strength of evidence for weight-related outcomes in studies taking place in a school setting with a home and consumer health informatics component

Setting	Intervention, n	Years of Publication	Enrolled Participants	Studies With Low/ Moderate/ High Risk of Bias(n)	% With Favorable (Statistically Sig) Outcome	% With Favorable Outcome (Does Not Need to be Stat Sig)	Risk of Bias	Consistency	Precision	Directness	Strength of the Evidence
School-Home-CHI	C,1	2011	589	0/0/1	0	0	High	NA	Imprecise	Direct	Insufficient

C = combination of diet and physical activity interventions; CHI = consumer health informatics; sig = significant

Key Question 2: What is the comparative effectiveness of home-based interventions for the prevention of obesity or overweight in children?

Key Points

Diet, physical activity and combination (diet and physical activity) interventions did not show any significant impact on weight-related outcomes and the evidence is low, at best, inconclusive that any of these interventions are more effective in preventing obesity or overweight than the control.

Home-Based Studies

Study Characteristics

We included four RCTs, and all were from the U.S.[171-174]Three of the studies reported that preventing obesity was the goal of the intervention.[171,173,174] One study included children greater than 5 years of age.[173] One study included only girls,[172] and two studies based inclusion criteria on a BMI less than the 85th percentile (Table 21; Appendix E, Evidence Table 29).[171,172]

Population Characteristics

The total number of participants in all four studies was 321. The total followup period ranged from 52[171,173] to 104 weeks.[172] In one study all of the participants were girls[172] and in two other studies[171,174] 50-65 percent of the participants were girls. The age range of the participants in all four studies was 4 to 17 years. Only one of the four studies reported the grade level and participants were preschoolers[174]. One of the four studies described the race of the participants.[174] In this study, 94 percent of the participants were Latin Hispanic, 2 percent Black non-Hispanic and 4 percent multiracial/other[174] (Table 21; Appendix E, Evidence Table 30).

Interventions

One of the four studies reported on an educational diet-only intervention.[172] This study evaluated the effect of a calcium-rich diet on weight gain among girls over a 104-week study period. Three of the four home-based studies examined the effect of a combined diet and physical activity intervention on weight outcomes. One of these three studies compared the effect on change in weight at 52 weeks of two educational diet and physical activity interventions, each addressing a different dietary behavior (increased fruit and vegetable intake vs. decreased intake of high fat/high sugar foods).[171] The second study[173] evaluated the effect of a 52-week combined diet and physical activity intervention on television viewing, snack/sweet intake, eating out, and physical activity among entire households. A third study[174] assessed the effect of a combined intervention on dietary fat, fruit and vegetable intake, television viewing, and physical activity. (Table 22; Appendix E, Evidence Table 31).

Table 21. Study and participant characteristics of studies based in the home

Author, Year	RCT	Goal: Obesity Prevention	Country	Sex*	Age Range, Years*	Grade*	Other	Total N	Followup in Weeks	% Girls†	Mean Age [Range] Years†	Grade†	Race†
Home													
Epstein, 2001[171]	Y	Y	U.S.	NR	6-11	NR		26	52	65	8.6-8.8	NR	NR
Fitzgibbon, 2012[174]	Y	Y	U.S.	NR	3-5	Pre-school		146	52	50	4.5	Pre-school	BNH 2 Latino 94 Other 4
French, 2011[173]	Y	Y	U.S.	NR	>5	NR		90 househ olds	52	NR	5-17	NR	NR
Lappe, 2004[172]	Y	N	U.S.	Girls	9	NR		59	104	100	9.5	NR	NR
Home/PC/CHI													
Patrick, 2006[175]	Y	N	U.S.	NR	11-15	NR		878	52	49.9	12.7	NR	WNH: 58.4 BNH: 6.6 Hispanic 13.1 API: 3.2 AIAN: 0.7 other: 18
Home/ School/ Community													
Gentile, 2009[176]	Y	Y	U.S.	NR	NR	3-5		1323	61	53	9.6	3-5	WNH: 90%

AIAN = American Indian/Alaska Native; API = Asian Pacific Islander; BMI = body mass index (in kg/m^2); BP = blood pressure; CHI = consumer health informatics; CVD = cardiovascular disease; Maint = maintenance; meds = medications; N = no; NR = not reported; PC = physical activity; PC = primary care; RCT = randomized controlled trials; WNH = White non-Hispanic; Y = yes

* Inclusion/exclusion criteria.
† Participant characteristics.

100

Table 22. Interventions of studies based in the home

Author, Year	Control Arm	Description of Intervention	Diet (Phys/Env)	Diet (Psych)	Physical Activity (Phys/Env)	Physical Activity (Psych)
		Home				
Epstein, 2001[171]	NA	Take home child workbook; active parental involvement (parent-focused intervention) to increase fruit and vegetable intake.		X		X
		Take home child workbook; active parental involvement (parent-focused intervention) to decrease fat and sugar intake.		X		X
Fitzgibbon, 2012[174]	Usual care	Nutrition instruction, combined with the physical activity component, was designed to target specific child behaviors. Creating a home environment to facilitate healthy choices. Interactive instruction on family exercise (and healthful eating). Classroom sessions included an aerobic activity component.	X	X	X	X
French, 2011[173]	Usual care	Education sessions to - limit consumption of high calorie, limit sweetened drinks, eat at least 5 servings fruits and vegetables each day, eat smaller portions ("eat less"), limit eating fast foods, make healthy choices when eating out. Provided guidelines on healthy choices. Sessions to encourage 30 minutes of activity per day.	X	X	X	X
Lappe, 2004[172]	Usual care	Eating calcium rich and fortified foods, no supplements		X		
		Home/PC/CHI				
Patrick, 2006[175]	Usual care	Computer-based counseling and brief provider counseling with a 16-section printed Teen Guide, mail, and telephone counseling to modify total intake of fat, servings per day of fruits and vegetables, physical activity, and sedentary behaviors.		X		X
		Home/ School/ Community				
Gentile, 2009[176]	Usual care	The Switch program promoted healthy active lifestyles by encouraging students to 'Switch what you Do (exercise), Chew (eat), and View (sedentary activity)'.		X		X

CHI = consumer health informatics; PC = primary care; Psych = psychosocial intervention; Phys/Env = physical/environmental intervention

101

Outcomes

Diet Interventions

One out of the four home-based studies was a diet intervention that enrolled 63 girls and randomized 59 to the intervention and control groups.[172]

Weight-Related Outcomes

BMI

There was no reported difference in BMI at 104 weeks between the intervention and control arms (Appendix E, Evidence Table 32a).[172]

Percent Body Fat

There was no reported difference in fat mass at 104 weeks between the intervention and control arms (Appendix E, Evidence Table 32a).[172]

Weight

There was no reported difference in weight at 104 weeks between the intervention and control arms (Appendix E, Evidence Table 32a).[172]

Clinical Outcomes

None reported.

Adverse Events

None reported.

Intermediate Outcomes

Physical Activity and Sedentary Behaviors

There was no difference in self-reported hours of physical activity between the intervention and control arms (Appendix E, Evidence Table 32b).[172]

Dietary Intake

At 104 weeks the intervention group had a higher total energy intake compared to the control group. The study did not statistically analyze this between group difference (Appendix E, Evidence Table 32b).[172]

Interpretation

We can make no conclusions on the effectiveness of a home-based diet intervention on obesity or overweight prevention. This is based on the results from a single diet intervention study. This study evaluated the effect of the intervention on BMI percent body fat and weight and found no significant between-group difference with respect to these outcomes. This study also reported on change in physical activity and energy intake and found no significant between-group difference with respect to these outcomes. The study did not specifically target weight gain prevention but rather the effects of a high-calcium diet on weight over a 104-week period. The intervention did not include other dietary modifications or physical activity components. All of the above mentioned factors may have contributed to the attenuated effect of the intervention on weight and intermediate outcomes. Additionally, a larger sample size may be necessary to further evaluate the impact of the intervention.

Physical Activity Intervention
None reported.

Diet and Physical Activity Intervention
Three of the four home-based studies evaluated the effects of combined diet and physical activity intervention on weight outcomes.[171,173,174] One study enrolled 30 families and randomized 26 children into two intervention groups.[171] Another study randomized 90 participating households with children aged 5-17 to intervention or control group for 52 weeks.[173] A third study consisted of 146 children randomly assigned to receive the intervention or control.[174]

Weight-Related Outcomes

BMI z-Score
Two home-based studies assessed the effect of a combined diet and physical activity intervention on BMI z-score. In both studies there was no significant intervention effect on BMI z-score at 52 weeks followup (p>0.05) (Appendix E, Evidence Table 33a).[173,174]

BMI
In one of these three studies, there was no significant between- group difference at the post-intervention or 1-year followup visit (p>0.05).[174] (Appendix E, Evidence Table 33a).[174]

Prevalence of Overweight and Obesity
At 52 weeks, one study demonstrated a decrease in the percent of overweight children in the increased fruit and vegetable group of 1.10 percent (S.D. 5.29), and a 2.40 (S.D. 5.39) percent decrease in percent of overweight children in the decreased high fat/high sugar intervention group. This difference was not statistically different (p>0.05).[171] A second study reported that the prevalence of obesity among all participants decreased from 21 to 15 percent at 52 weeks. The study did not report or statistically analyze this change by intervention or control group. (Appendix E, Evidence Table 33a).

Weight
In one study there was no significant intervention effect on weight post-intervention or at the 52-week followup period (p value>0.05) (Appendix E, Evidence Table 33a).[171]

Clinical Outcomes
None reported.

Adverse Events
None reported.

Intermediate Outcomes

Physical Activity and Sedentary Behavior

In two studies there was no significant difference between the intervention and control group in minutes per day of physical activity (Appendix E, Evidence Table 33b).[173,174]

In two studies there was no significant difference between the intervention and control group in TV viewing or general screen time (Appendix E, Evidence Table 33b)[173,174]

Dietary Intake

All three studies[171,173,174] demonstrated a favorable intervention effect on fruit and vegetable intake but only one study[173] demonstrated a statistically significant intervention effect on fruit and vegetable intake among adolescents only (p=0.05) (Appendix E, Evidence Table 33b).[173]

In one study there was no difference in sugar-sweetened beverage intake between the intervention and control group (p=0.96)(Appendix E, Evidence Table 33b).[173]

In another study there was no difference between the intervention and control in energy intake (Appendix E, Evidence Table 33b).[174]

Interpretation

The strength of the evidence is low that combined diet and physical activity interventions in a home setting effectively prevent obesity or overweight. Combined interventions in this setting had a beneficial effect on fruit and vegetable intake. However, no conclusions can be made regarding their effect on other dietary, physical activity, or sedentary behaviors. These conclusions are supported by results of three studies reporting on the effect of combined diet and physical activity interventions in the home setting.[171,173,174]

One study reported on BMI and did not demonstrate a favorable or significant intervention effect with respect to this outcome measure.[174] Another study reported on BMI z-score and did not demonstrate a statistically significant or favorable intervention effect.[173] A third study reported on prevalence of overweight and demonstrated a change in favor of one intervention group.[171] This change in prevalence of overweight was not statistically significant.[171]

Two studies reported on physical activity and sedentary behavior.[173,174] Both studies demonstrated a favorable but nonsignificant intervention effect on physical activity.[173,174] Neither study demonstrated a favorable or significant intervention effect on screen time.[173,174]

Three studies demonstrated a favorable intervention effect on fruit and vegetable intake;[171,173,174] one of these was significant[173] and two were not significant.[171,173] One study reported on sugar-sweetened beverages and did not demonstrate a favorable or significant intervention effect.[173] One study reported on energy intake and did not demonstrate a favorable or significant intervention effect.[174]

Use of interventions with significant parental/family involvement may have contributed to beneficial intervention effects studies demonstrated on select intermediate outcomes. However, additional studies with larger sample sizes, greater intervention intensity and longer followup may be necessary to further evaluate the impact of combined home based interventions on the prevention of obesity in children.

Strength of the Evidence

Weight-Related Outcomes

No conclusion can be made about the effectiveness of a home-based diet intervention on obesity prevention. We based this on a single study with moderate risk of bias and no measurable impact of the intervention. The strength of evidence is low that combined diet and physical activity interventions in a home setting positively impact obesity prevention. We graded the strength of evidence low because it included three moderate to high risk of bias studies, that were inconsistent (one demonstrated a positive effect, two demonstrated a negative effect) and imprecise (Table 23, Appendix F, Strength of Evidence Table 1).

Intermediate Outcomes

No conclusion can be made about the effectiveness of combined diet and physical activity interventions in a home setting on physical activity, screen time, sugar-sweetened beverage intake or energy intake. We graded this body of evidence as insufficient because it included inconsistent studies with moderate to high risk of bias and imprecise results. The strength of the evidence is low that combined diet and physical activity interventions in a home setting positively impact fruit and vegetable intake. This is due to the moderate risk of bias, consistent effect in favor of the intervention, and lack of precision (Appendix F, Strength of Evidence Tables 2, 4-7).

Table 23. Summary of the strength of evidence for weight-related outcomes in studies taking place in a home setting

Setting	Intervention, n	Years of Publication	Enrolled Participants	Studies With Low/Mode Rate/High Risk of Bias(n)	% With Favorable (Statistically Sig) Outcome	% With Favorable Outcome (Does Not Need to be Stat Sig)	Risk of Bias	Consistency	Precision	Directness	Strength of the Evidence
Home	D, 1	2004	59	0/1/0	0	0	Moderate	NA	Imprecise	Direct	Insufficient
	C, 3	2001-2012	262	0/2/1	0	33	Moderate	Inconsistent	Imprecise	Direct	Low

D = diet intervention; PA = physical activity intervention; C = combination of diet and physical activity interventions

106

Home-Primary Care-Consumer Health Informatics–Based Studies

Study Characteristics

We included one RCT conducted in the U.S.[175]. The study's stated goal was to improve diet, physical activity and sedentary behaviors.[175] The study included participants aged 11 to 15 years, and participants who did not have health conditions which could have limited their ability to comply with physical activity or diet recommendations (Table 21; Appendix E, Evidence Table 34).[175]

Population Characteristics

The study included a total of 878 participants.[175] The total followup period was 52 weeks. Forty nine percent were girls and the mean age of all participants was 12.7 years (+/- 1.3 years.) The study did not report the grade level of the participants.[175] In this study[175] 58.4 percent of participants were white, 6.6 percent African-American, 13.1 percent Hispanic, 3.2 percent Asian or Pacific Islander, 0.7 percent Native American, and 18 percent multi-ethnic or other (Table 21; Appendix E, Evidence Table 35).

Interventions

This study reported on a 52-week educational diet and physical activity intervention.[175] The study evaluated how a multi-strategy intervention (computer-supported assessment followed by provider counseling [monthly mail and telephone counseling]) affected eating and physical activity behaviors (Table 22; Appendix E, Evidence Table 36).

Outcomes

Diet Interventions

None reported.

Physical Activity Interventions

None reported.

Diet and Physical Activity Interventions

One study evaluated the effects of a combined diet and physical activity intervention relative to a control group on BMI z-score at 52 weeks.[175] The study randomized 878 participants and included 819 in the analysis.

Weight-Related Outcomes

BMI z-Score

The study reported no significant difference in overall BMI z score at 52 weeks between the intervention and control arms ($p \geq 0.05$) (Appendix E, Evidence Table 37a).[175] Among participants with a BMI greater than or equal to the 95th percentile, mean BMI z-score was 0.04 less in the intervention group compared to the control group at 52 weeks, which was not statistically significantly different ($p=0.10$)[175] (Appendix E, Evidence Table 37a,b).

Clinical Outcomes
None reported.

Adverse Events
None reported

Intermediate Outcomes

Physical Activity and Sedentary Activity
The study reported no significant difference in minutes per week of moderate plus vigorous physical activity between the intervention and control group among girls (p=0.90) or boys (p=0.017)(Appendix E, Evidence Table 37c).[175]

The number of hours per day of sedentary behaviors decreased significantly in the intervention group compared to the control at 52 weeks among girls and boys (p=0.001) (Appendix E, Evidence Table 37c).[175]

Dietary Intake
The study reported no significant difference in percent calories from fat among girls (p=0.86) or boys (p=0.31), nor in fruit and vegetable consumption between the intervention and control groups among girls (p=0.07) or boys (p=0.49) (Appendix E, Evidence Table 37c).

Interpretation
We can make no conclusions regarding the effectiveness of a combined diet and physical activity intervention in a home setting with primary care and consumer health informatics components on obesity or overweight. No conclusions can be made regarding the effectiveness of a combined diet and physical activity intervention in a home setting with primary care and consumer health informatics components on diet and physical activity. Combined diet and physical activity interventions in this setting have a favorable and significant effect on sedentary behaviors. We based this on results of a single study reporting on a combined diet and physical activity intervention.[175]

This study evaluated the effect of an intervention on BMI z-score.[175] and reported a favorable but nonstatistically significant intervention effect on BMI z-score among obese adolescents[175] and a nonsignificant intervention effect on BMI z-score for the overall sample.[175] We were unable to determine if there was a favorable effect of the intervention because the study did not provide BMI z-score values for the overall sample. This study demonstrated a favorable and statistically significant intervention effect on sedentary behaviors and demonstrated a favorable but nonsignificant intervention effect on physical activity among boys[175] and a favorable but nonsignificant intervention effect on fruit and vegetable intake among girls.[175]

The integrated approach, including family engagement, computer-based behavioral assessments, and provider and telephone counseling, may have contributed to observed beneficial effects on select intermediate outcomes. However, additional studies with longer followup and greater intervention intensity may be needed to appreciate subsequent changes in weight-related outcomes.

Strength of the Evidence

Weight-Related Outcomes

We make no conclusions regarding the effectiveness of a combined diet and physical activity intervention in a home setting with primary care and consumer health informatics components on obesity or overweight. This is due to the inclusion of a single study that lacked precision with regard to the results from the overall sample. We were unable to determine the magnitude of the intervention effect on BMI z-score for the entire sample because the study did not provide actual outcome values (Table 24; Appendix F, Strength of Evidence Table 1).

Intermediate Outcomes

We can make no conclusions regarding the effectiveness of a combined diet and physical activity intervention in a home setting with primary care and consumer health informatics components on diet or physical activity. This was due to the inclusion of a single study that lacked precision and demonstrated favorable effect for sex-based subgroups only. The strength of evidence is low that a combined diet and physical activity intervention in a home setting with primary care and consumer health informatics components positively impacts sedentary behaviors. This is due to the low risk of bias, favorable effect on the outcome for the overall sample and high precision (Appendix F, Strength of Evidence Tables, 2,4,6, and 7).

Table 24. Summary of the strength of evidence for weight-related outcomes in studies taking place in a home setting with primary care and consumer health informatics components

Setting	Intervention, n	Years of Publication	Enrolled Participants	Studies With Low/ Moderate/ High Risk of Bias(n)	% With Favorable (Statistically Sig) Outcome	% With Favorable Outcome (Does Not Need to be Stat Sig)	Risk of Bias	Consistency	Precision	Directness	Strength of the Evidence
Home-PC-CHI	C, 1	2006	878	1/0/0	0	Unable to determine – actual outcome values not reported only significance	Low	NA	Imprecise	Direct	Insufficient

C = combination diet and physical activity intervention; PC = primary care; CHI = consumer health informatics; NA = not applicable

110

Home-School-Community–Based Studies

Study Characteristics

We included one RCT conducted in the U.S.[176] The stated goal of the intervention was to prevent obesity. Participants included students attending grade 3 through 5 of two community school districts (Table 21; Appendix E, Evidence Table 38).

Population Characteristics

The study included a total of 1,323 participants. The total followup period (including an additional measurement period at 6 months post-intervention) was 61 weeks. Roughly half (53 percent) of the participants were girls. The mean age of the participants was 9.6 (+/- 0.9 years). All of participants were in grades 3 through 5 and 90 percent of participants were white (Table 21; Appendix E, Evidence Table 39).

Interventions

This study reported on an educational diet and physical activity intervention. It evaluated the effects of the intervention on three targeted behaviors (increase fruit and vegetable intake, increase physical activity, and decreased screen time) over a 61-week study period (Table 22; Appendix E, Evidence Table 40).

Outcomes

Diet Intervention

None reported.

Physical Activity Intervention

None reported.

Diet and Physical Activity Intervention Studies

One study evaluated the effects of a combined diet and physical activity intervention relative to a control group on BMI at 34 and 61 weeks.[176] The study randomized 1,323 participants and included 992 in the analysis at all three data collection points (baseline, post intervention, and 6 months post intervention).

Weight-Related Outcomes

BMI

At 34 weeks, mean BMI was 19 kg/m^2 (S.E. 0.03) for the control group, and 19 kg/m^2 (S.E. 0.02) for the intervention group. The difference in mean BMI between the groups did not reach statistical significance ($p \geq 0.06$) (Evidence Table 41a). At 61 weeks, the mean BMI was 19.5 kg/m^2 (S.E. 0.1) for the control group and 19.4 kg/m^2 (S.E. 0.1) for the intervention group. The difference in mean BMI between the groups did not reach statistical significance ($p \geq 0.05$) (Appendix E, Evidence Table 41a).

There was a significant effect difference in boys at 61 weeks ($p < 0.05$), with boys in the intervention group demonstrating a 0.3 kg/m2 lower BMI than boys in the control group (Evidence Table 41b).

Clinical Outcomes

None reported.

Adverse Events

None reported.

Intermediate Outcomes

Physical Activity and Sedentary Activity

There was no statistically significant difference in physical activity (steps/day) or screen time between the intervention and control group at either followup time period (Appendix E, Evidence Table 41c).

Dietary Intake

Children in the intervention group reported significantly more fruit and vegetable consumption compared to the control group at 61 weeks (p<0.05). (Appendix E, Evidence Table 41c).

Interpretation

We can make no conclusions regarding the effectiveness of a combined diet and physical activity intervention in a home setting with school and community components on obesity or overweight. We can make no conclusions regarding the effectiveness of a combined diet and physical activity intervention in a home setting with school and community components on diet, physical activity, or sedentary behaviors. This is due to the results of a single study reporting on a combined diet and physical activity intervention.[176]

This study evaluated the effect of the intervention on BMI and found no favorable or statistically significant effect for the overall sample. However, it demonstrated a significant intervention effect among boys at 61 weeks.[176] This study also reported on the effect of the intervention on child-reported physical activity, screen time, and fruit and vegetable intake and demonstrated a favorable effect with respect to these outcome measures at 61 weeks. However, only fruit and vegetable intake was significantly different between the intervention and control groups at 61 weeks.

A comprehensive approach with family, school, and community components, may have contributed to observed beneficial effects on behavior change. However, additional studies of greater quality with longer intervention duration and followup may be needed to appreciate subsequent changes in weight-related outcomes.

Strength of the Evidence

Weight-Related Outcomes

We can make no conclusions regarding the effectiveness of a combined diet and physical activity intervention in a home setting with school and community components on obesity or overweight. This is due to the inclusion of a single study with high risk of bias, and poor precision with respect to BMI for the overall sample (Table 25; Appendix F, Strength of Evidence Table 1).

Intermediate Outcomes

We can make no conclusions regarding the effectiveness of a combined diet and physical activity intervention in a home setting with school and community components on diet, physical activity or sedentary behaviors. This is due to the inclusion of a single study with high risk of bias (Appendix F, Strength of Evidence Tables 4, 6, and 7).

Table 25. Summary of the strength of evidence for weight-related outcomes in studies taking place in a home setting with school and community components

Setting	Intervention, n	Years of Publication	Enrolled Participants	Studies With Low/ Moderate/ High Risk of Bias(n)	% With Favorable (Statistically Sig) Outcome	% With Favorable Outcome (Does Not Need to be Stat Sig)	Risk of Bias	Consistency	Precision	Directness	Strength of the Evidence
Home-School-Community	C, 1	2009	1323	0/0/1	0	0	High	NA	Imprecise	Direct	Insufficient

C = combination diet and physical activity intervention; NA = not applicable

Key Question 3: What is the comparative effectiveness of primary care-based interventions for the prevention of obesity or overweight in children?

Key Points

We can make no conclusions regarding the effectiveness of a combined diet and physical activity intervention in a primary care setting on obesity or overweight prevention.

Primary Care–Based Studies

Study Characteristics

We included one study from the U.S. that used a quasi-experimental design.[177] The goal of the intervention was to prevent obesity. The study included participants aged 5 to 18 years (Table 26; Appendix E, Evidence Table 42).

Population Characteristics

The study included 600 subjects[177]. The followup period was 78 weeks,[177] 47 percent of participants were girls, 56 percent were 5-11 years, and 44 percent were 12-17 years. This study did not report race or grade level (Table 26; Appendix E, Evidence Table 43).[178]

Interventions

One study[177] reported on a combined diet and physical activity intervention and used educational and physical environmental approaches including improving clinical decision support, counseling families and patients on "5-2-1-0" behavioral goals (consuming at least five or more servings of fruits and vegetables daily, limiting screen time to no more than 2 hours daily, engaging in at least 1 hour or more of daily physical activity, and avoiding sugar-sweetened beverages), and providing overall practice and provider management over the entire 78-week study period (Table 27; Appendix E, Evidence Table 44).

Table 26. Summary table for study and participant characteristics in primary-care based settings

Author, Year	RCT	Goal: Obesity Prevention	Country	Sex*	Age Range, Years*	Grade*	Other*	Total N	Followup in Weeks	% Girls[†]	Mean Age [Range] Years[†]	Grade[†]	Race[†]
Polacsek, 2009[177]	N	Y	U.S.	NR	5-18 years	NR	NR	600	78	47	5-17 years	NR	NR

N = no; NR = not reported; RCT = randomized controlled trials; Y = yes
*Inclusion/exclusion criteria.
[†]Participant characteristics.

Table 27. Summary table for intervention in primary care-based settings

Author, Year	Control Arm	Description of Intervention	Diet (Phys/Env)	Diet (Psych)	Physical Activity (Phys/Env)	Physical Activity (Psych)
Polacsek, 2009[177]	NA	Encouraging >5 servings of fruits and vegetables daily; limiting screen time to <2 hours daily and; avoiding (0) sugar-sweetened beverages and greater than 1 hour of physical activity daily. Pediatric Obesity Clinical Decision Support Chart with an algorithm and guidelines for the prevention and management of overweight.	X	X	X	X

Psych = psychosocial intervention; Phys/Env = physical/environmental intervention; NA = not applicable

116

Outcomes

Diet Interventions
None reported

Physical Activity Interventions
None reported.

Diet and Physical Activity Interventions
One non-RCT study included 600 participants in the analysis.[177]

Prevalence of Overweight and Obesity
The prevalence of overweight in the intervention group increased from 36.8 to 38.9 percent during the study. The study did not statistically analyze this change (Appendix E, Evidence Table 45a).[177] The prevalence of obesity in the intervention group increased from 19.8 to 20.3 percent during the study. The study did not statistically analyze this change (Appendix E, Evidence Table 45a).[177]

Clinical Outcomes
None reported.

Adverse Events
None reported.

Intermediate Outcomes

Physical Activity and Sedentary Activity
Fifteen percent of parents reported making physical activity changes for themselves and their children (Appendix E, Evidence Table 45b).[177] The study did not measure parent-reported behavioral changes at baseline.

Twelve percent of parents reported making TV/screen changes for themselves and their children (Appendix E, Evidence Table 45b).[177] The study did not measure parent-reported behavioral changes at baseline.

Dietary Intake
In the study, 26 percent of parents reported making nutrition changes and 17 percent of parents reported making changes in sugar-sweetened beverages consumption for themselves and their children (Appendix E, Evidence Table 45b).[177] The study did not measure parent-reported behavioral changes at baseline.

Interpretation
We can make no conclusions regarding the effectiveness of a combined diet and physical activity intervention in a primary care setting on obesity or overweight. We can make no conclusions regarding the effectiveness of a combined diet and physical activity intervention in a primary care setting on diet, physical activity or sedentary behaviors. This is due to the results of a single arm study reporting on a combined diet and physical activity intervention.[177] This study

evaluated the effect of an intervention on prevalence of overweight and obesity, both of which increased during the intervention. The study did not statistically analyze this change in prevalence of overweight and obesity. The study reported on percent of parents reporting diet, physical activity and screen time changes, based on surveys conducted during the intervention. However, it did not report any baseline values for these outcomes, hence we could not fully assess the intervention effect. Although the study's overall goal was to reduce the risk of childhood obesity, the intervention primarily aimed to achieve this goal through direct improvement of clinical decision support and family management of risk behaviors. Hence the intervention effect on weight outcomes may have been attenuated. Additional factors that may have limited intervention effectiveness include the lack of randomization, absent comparison group, and failure to reassess weight outcomes following the completion of the intervention. Parental reports of behavior changes did not appear to impact their children's outcomes.

Strength of the Evidence

Weight-Related Outcomes

We can make no conclusions regarding the effectiveness of a combined diet and physical activity intervention in a primary care setting on obesity or overweight prevention. This is due to the inclusion of a single imprecise study with a moderate risk of bias (Table 28, Appendix F, Strength of Evidence Table 1).

Intermediate Outcomes

We can make no conclusions regarding the effectiveness of a combined diet and physical activity intervention in a primary care setting on diet, physical activity or sedentary behaviors. This is due to the inclusion of a single imprecise study with a moderate risk of bias and no testable intervention effect (Appendix F, Strength of Evidence Tables 6 and 7).

Table 28. Summary of the strength of evidence for weight-related outcomes in studies taking place in a primary care setting

Setting	Intervention, n	Years of Publication	Enrolled Participants	Studies With Low/ Moderate/ High Risk of Bias(n)	% With Favorable (Statistically Sig) Outcome	% With Favorable Outcome (Does Not Need to be Stat Sig)	Risk of Bias	Consistency	Precision	Directness	Strength of the Evidence
Primary Care	C, 1	2009	600	0/1/0	0	0	Moderate	NA	Imprecise	Direct	Insufficient

C = combination diet and physical activity intervention; NA = not applicable

119

Key Question 4: What is the comparative effectiveness of child-care-based interventions for the prevention of obesity or overweight in children?

Key Points

One non-RCT study tested an educational physical activity intervention and found significant differences in weight outcomes between the intervention and control groups. The strength of evidence is insufficient that diet alone or physical activity alone prevent obesity or overweight in child-care setting.

Two out of three studies showed no statistical difference in weight outcomes between the intervention and control groups. Combined diet and physical activity interventions implemented in child-care setting showed no beneficial effect at preventing obesity, with a low strength of evidence.

Childcare–Based Studies

Study Characteristics

Five articles reported on four studies.[77,102,179,180] Two articles[77,181] reported on one study and count as one study. Three were RCTs[77,179,180] and one was a non-randomized[102] prospective study. Two[77,180] out of the four studies conducted in child-care settings stated the goal of the study was obesity prevention and weight maintenance in children. Only one study[180] took place in the U.S., while two[102,179] took place in Germany and one in Switzerland[77] (Table 29; Appendix E, Evidence Table 46).

Population Characteristics

The number of participants in four included studies was 2,657. The followup period for one was 52 weeks,[77] for another was 78 weeks[179] and for two others was 104 weeks.[102,180] Across all studies 47.6 to 50 percent of the participants were girls. The age range of the participants in all four studies was 3 to 6.1 years. Two out of the four studies reported the grade level and participants in both studies were preschoolers.[77,102] Only one study described race and the race distribution was as follows: 81.4 percent Hispanic, 11.5 percent Black, and 7.5 percent others/multiracial[180] (Table 29; Appendix E, Evidence Table 47).

Interventions

One study reported on a physical activity intervention comprising of a playful-athletic exercise program lasting 1 hour, 3 times a week.[102] The exercises were easy to do and included running with a newspaper in front of the breast without letting the paper fall down, jumping from a chalk circle into another and balancing on a line. This non-RCT evaluated the effect of 104 weeks of physical activity training on BMI, percent body fat, and skinfold thickness in pre-school children in 17 nursery schools in Berlin.

Three studies[77,179,180] evaluated the effect of combined diet and physical activity interventions. One of them included an educational component and alterations in food served and physical activity recommended during an aftercare program for kindergarteners.[179] It aimed to achieve this through educating care providers and communication with families. The study analyzed two samples, control and intervention, containing different children, at time intervals of 5.7 and 17.6 months after the start of the intervention.[179]

Another study randomized 12 Latino Head Start centers to a culturally tailored combined diet and physical activity intervention or control group.[180] The intervention consisted of a variety of diet and physical activity modification curriculum delivered by trained early childhood educators for 14 weeks. This included 20 minutes of nutritional activity based on hand puppets reflecting the food pyramid and 20 minutes of aerobic activity. Behaviors for the intervention included increased fruit and vegetable consumption, decreased fat intake, decreased sedentary behaviors, and increased physical activity.

The third study had a multidimensional culturally tailored intervention which included a physical activity program, lessons on nutrition, media use, and sleep for pre-school children in a high migrant population.[77] (Table 30; Appendix E, Evidence Table 48).

Table 29. Study and participant characteristics of studies based in childcare settings

Author, Year	RCT	Goal: Obesity Prevention	Country	Sex*	Age Range, Years*	Grade*	Other*	Total N	Followup in Weeks	% Girls†	Mean Age [Range] Years†	Grade†	Race†
Bayer, 2009[179]	Y	N	Germany	NR	NR	NR	NR	1,340	78	47.6	6.12	Kindergarten	NR
Fitzgibbon, 2006[180]	Y	Y	U.S.	NR	NR	NR	NR	401	104	49.4	4.3	Pre-school	Latino 81.4% Black 11.5% Other 7.5%
Metcalf, 2012[77] Burgi 2012[181]	Y	Y	Switzerland	NR	NR	Pre School	NR	652	52	50	5.2	Pre-school	NR
Scheffler, 2007[102]	N	N	Germany	NR	NR	Pre School	NR	264	104	NR	NR	NR	NR

N = no; NR = not reported; RCT = randomized controlled trials; Y = yes
*Inclusion/exclusion criteria.
†Participant characteristics.

122

Table 30. Interventions of studies based in child-care settings

Author, Year	Control Arm	Description of Intervention	Diet (Phys/Env)	Diet (Psych)	Physical Activity (Phys/Env)	Physical Activity (Psych)
Bayer, 2009[179]	Usual care	Tiger Kids "low cost behavioral intervention." An Internet platform with supporting information for Kindergarten teachers and families: modifying habits of food and drink consumption, and regular consumption of water and other nonsugared drinks. Offer fruits and vegetables throughout the day. Information materials and modules with songs for use in the day care Enhancing physical activity.	X	X	X	X
Fitzgibbon, 2006[180]	Usual care	Nutrition activity based on hand puppets that reflected the food pyramid. Curriculum to increase physical activity and aerobic activity.	X		X	
Metcalf, 2012[77] Burgi, 2012[181]	Usual care	Information sessions for children focusing on healthy nutrition. Information sessions that included promoting physical activity. Extra physical activity sessions, additional exercise equipment was provided.	X	X	X	X
Scheffler, 2007[102]	Usual care	Playful athletic exercise programs were designed. The exercises targeted improving the pleasure of movement and train the motor basics like endurance, power, speed and skillfulness.				X

Psych = psychosocial intervention; Phys/Env = physical/environmental intervention

123

Outcomes

Diet Interventions

No study reported.

Physical Activity Interventions

One study out of the four child-care center-based studies was a physical activity intervention that enrolled 264 children from 17 nursery schools and followed them for 104 weeks.[102]

Weight-Related Outcomes

BMI

The study reported an increase in the BMI of intervention children compared with children of the control group in both sexes (16.56 kg/m^2 vs. 16.41 kg/m^2 in boys and 16.10 kg/m^2 vs. 15.86 kg/m^2 in girls, no p value reported).[102] However with the additional analysis of body composition (e.g., skeleton, body fat) the data indicates that the comparative high BMI in the physical activity intervention group is a result of higher percentage of muscle and not body fat[102] (Appendix E, Evidence Table 49a).

Percent Body Fat

Similarly this study reported a significant lower percentage of body fat in the intervention group compared to the control group (16.34 vs. 17.26 percent in boys and 19.33 vs. 19.75 percent in girls, no p value reported)[102] (Appendix E, Evidence Table 49a).

Skinfold Thickness

This study also reported a significant decrease in triceps skinfold thickness in the intervention group compared to the control group (8.05 mm vs. 8.64 mm in boys and 9.10 vs. 9.26 in girls, no p value reported)[102] (Appendix E, Evidence Table 49a).

Clinical Outcomes

The physical activity-only intervention resulted in significant lower diastolic blood pressure at 104 weeks after the start of the intervention (Intervention group 62.0 SD 11.2 mm Hg vs. 68.8 SD 11.1 mm Hg, $p<0.001$) (Appendix E, Evidence Table 49b).

Adverse Events

None reported.

Intermediate Outcomes

None reported.

Interpretation

The results from an outcome measure from the one study reporting on physical activity interventions in a child-care setting support our conclusions. In this study, there was no significant beneficial physical activity intervention effect on BMI but there were significant positive intervention effect with respect to percent body fat, skinfold thickness, and diastolic blood pressure in a child-care setting. We need more well-designed studies to further evaluate the impact of the intervention in this setting.

Diet and Physical Activity Intervention

Three RCTs out of the four child-care center-based studies assessed the effects of combined diet and physical activity diet on weight outcomes. One study randomly assigned 64 kindergartens as intervention or control with samples of 1,318 and 1,340 included in analyses[179]. Another study randomized 420 children attending 12 head start centers and followed them for 104 weeks. The third study randomized 652 children in a high migrant population.

Weight-Related Outcomes

BMI z-Score

One study reported on BMI z-score and found no significant difference between the intervention and control group at 52 weeks (0.00 vs. 0.07, p=0.56) and 104 weeks (-0.13 vs. 0.00, p=0.34) post intervention[180] (Appendix E, Evidence Table 50a,b).

BMI

Two studies reported on BMI and found no significant difference in BMI of intervention group compared with the control group. In one study the mean increase in BMI was 0.33 kg/m^2 versus 0.48 kg/m^2 (p =0.46) at 52 weeks and 0.46 kg/m^2 vs. 0.70 kg/m^2 (p =0.34) at 104 weeks followup.[180] The second study reported that compared with the control children in the intervention group had no significant difference in BMI (-0.07 kg/m^2, -0.19 to 0.06, p=0.31)[77](Appendix E, Evidence Table 50a,b).

Prevalence of Overweight and Obesity

Two studies reported on the prevalence of overweight and found no difference in the prevalence of overweight.[77,179] One study at 78 weeks followup found no difference between the intervention and the control groups.[179] The odds ratio for overweight was 0.73 (95% CI 0.51-1.04), p=0.054 in the first sample and 0.89 (95% CI 0.66-1.22), p=0.59 in the second sample.[179] Similarly, this study did not report any difference in the prevalence of obesity at 78 weeks between the intervention and the control groups. The odds ratio for obesity was 0.58 (95% CI 0.31-1.10), p=0.074 in the first sample and 0.79 (95% CI 0.35-1.77), p=0.63 in the second sample.[179] The second study found no difference between intervention (10.5 to 11.0 percent) and control group (13.0 to 14.9 percent) at 52 weeks post intervention (p=0.23)[77] (Appendix E, Evidence Table 50a,b).

Percent Body Fat

One study reported significant intervention effect on percent body fat. The percent body fat decreased from a baseline of 23.7 to 23.2 percent, 52 weeks post intervention in the intervention group and increased from 23.6 to 24.1 percent in the control group with a between group difference of -1.1, 95% CI-2.02 to -0.20 (p= 0.02)[77] (Appendix E, Evidence Table 50a,b).

Waist Circumference

The same study reported on and also found significant intervention effect on waist circumference. The waist circumference increased from a baseline of 52.8cm to 53.3cm, 52 weeks post intervention in the intervention group and increased from 52.8cm to 54.3cm in the control group with a between-group difference of -1.0, 95% CI-1.6 to -0.42 (p= 0.001)[77] (Appendix E, Evidence Table 50a,b).

Clinical Outcomes
None reported.

Adverse Events
None reported.

Intermediate Outcomes

Physical Activity and Sedentary Activity
Two combined diet and physical activity intervention studies reported on physical activity and neither found significant intervention effect[77,180] (Appendix E, Evidence Table 50c).

Dietary Intake
One combined diet and physical activity intervention resulted in higher fruit and vegetable consumption in the two different samples at 78 weeks after the start of the intervention compared to the control group. The odds ratio for high fruit consumption was 1.64 (95% CI 1.26-2.12), p<0.001 in the first sample and 1.59 (95% CI 1.26-2.01), p<0.001 in the second sample.[179] Another combined diet and physical intervention study found no significant intervention effect on total fat intake or fiber intake[180] (Appendix E, Evidence Table 50c).

Interpretation
The results from an outcome measure from three studies reporting on combined diet and physical activity interventions in a child-care setting support our conclusions. Across all three combined diet and physical activity intervention studies in the child-care center-based settings, there were no significant between-group differences with respect to BMI z-score,[180] BMI,[77] and prevalence of obesity and overweight.[179] One out of the three combined diet and physical activity intervention studies found significant increase in fruit and vegetable intake. However, none of these studies found significant intervention effect on physical activity, total fat intake, or fiber intake. The small sample size and poor quality of these studies may have contributed to the attenuated effect of the intervention on weight outcomes. We need high quality studies with a larger sample size to further evaluate the impact of the intervention.

Strength of the Evidence

Weight-Related Outcomes
The strength of evidence is insufficient that a physical activity intervention reduces BMI, percent body fat, and skinfold thickness in a child-care center-based (only) setting because only one study with high risk of bias and direct and imprecise results evaluated this intervention on the prevention of obesity. There is no evidence of benefit for combined diet and physical activity interventions delivered in a child-care setting for prevention of child overweight and obesity. The strength of evidence is low because studies that addressed these outcomes had moderate risk of bias with direct, consistent, and imprecise results (Table 31, Appendix F, Strength of Evidence Table 1).

Intermediate Outcomes

There is no evidence of benefit for combined diet and physical activity intervention based in a child-care setting on increasing physical activity among children. The confidence in this conclusion is low because studies evaluating these outcomes had moderate risk of bias with direct and consistent results. We could not make a conclusion about the effectiveness of combined diet and physical activity interventions on increasing dietary intake of fruits and vegetables, total fat intake or fiber intake in a child-care setting. The strength of evidence is insufficient that a combined diet and physical activity intervention increases the intake of fruits and vegetables, total fat intake, or fiber intake in a child-care center-based (only) setting because only one study with moderate risk of bias and precise result addressed these outcomes (Appendix F, Strength of Evidence Tables 2-4).

Table 31. Summary of the strength of evidence for weight-related outcomes in studies taking place in childcare

Setting	Intervention, n	Years of Publication	Enrolled Participants	Studies With Low/ Moderate/ High Risk of Bias(n)	% With favorable (Statistically Sig) Outcome	% With Favorable Outcome (Does Not Need to be Stat Sig)	Risk of Bias	Consistency	Precision	Directness	Strength of the Evidence
Childcare	P, 1	2007	268	0/0/1	100	100	High	NA	Precise	Direct	Insufficient
	C, 3	2009-2012	2393	1/2/0	33	33	Moderate	Inconsistent	Imprecise	Direct	Low

P = physical activity interventions; C = combination diet and physical activity interventions; NA = not applicable

128

Key Question 5: What is the comparative effectiveness of community-based or environment-level interventions for the prevention of obesity or overweight in children?

Key Points

Community and Community Plus–Based Studies

The strength of evidence is insufficient that a physical activity-only intervention is more effective at preventing obesity or overweight than the control based on one RCT study. We found positive but nonsignificant changes in percent body fat in this intervention.

The strength of evidence is moderate that a diet and physical activity intervention combined with other approaches is more effective at preventing obesity or overweight than the control based on six RCTs and two non-RCTs. We found desirable changes in BMI or BMI z-score in five of the nine studies.

Community-Only–Based Studies

Study Characteristics

One RCT took place in Switzerland. The stated goal of this study was not weight maintenance. This study included only boys participating in sports (Table 32; Appendix E, Evidence Table 51).[182]

Population Characteristics

The study included 46 participants and followed them for 52 weeks. All participants were middle school-aged. It did to report race (Table 32; Appendix E, Evidence Table 52).[182]

Interventions

The study included a combined diet and physical activity intervention (Table 33; Appendix E, Evidence Table 53).

Table 32. Study and participant characteristics of studies based in the community

Author, Year	RCT	Goal: Obesity Prevention	Country	Sex*	Age Range, Years*	Grade*	Other*	Total N	Followup in Weeks	% Girls[†]	Mean Age [Range] Years[†]	Grade[†]	Race[†]
Community Only													
Eiholzer, 2010[182]	Y	N	Switzerland	Boys	NR	NR	NR	46	52	0	13.3	NR	NR
Community/ School													
Sallis, 2003[75]	Y	Y	U.S.	NR	NR	NR	NR	24 schools (mean enrollment 1,109)	104	49	NR	NR	WNH: 39.5
Singh, 2009[183]	Y	Y	Nether-lands	NR	NR	NR	NR	1,108	32-80	53.3	12.7	NR	NR
Chomitz, 2010[184]	N	Y	U.S.	NR	>5	NR	NR	1,858	156	48.2	7.7	NR	WNH : 37.1 BNH: 37.3 Latino/Hispanic: 14.0 API: 10.2 Other: 1.7
Community/ School/ Home													
Economos, 2007[185]	N	Y	U.S.	NR	NR	NR	NR	1,178	43	NR	7.34 – 7.9	1st grade 32.2% -47.4% 2nd grade 23.7% -29.6% 3rd grade 28.9%-38.2%	WNH:37.8 – 51.7 BNH : 6.9 – 25.1 Latino/ Hispanic: 11.8 – 22.8 API : 2.3 – 9.1 Other: 11-23

130

Table 32. Study and participant characteristics of studies based in the community (continued)

Author, Year	RCT	Goal: Obesity Prevention	Country	Sex*	Age Range, Years*	Grade*	Other*	Total N	Followup in Weeks	% Girls[†]	Mean Age [Range] Years[†]	Grade[†]	Race[†]
Community/ Home													
Robinson, 2010[186]	Y	Y	U.S.	Girls	8-10	NR	NR	261	104	100	9.4	NR	BNH: 100%
Klesges, 2012[187]	Y	Y	U.S.	Girls	8-10	NR	BMI >= the 25th pctl, or < BMI – 35 or at least 1 parent with a BMI >r than 25	303	104	100	9.3	NR	African-American: 100
Community/ Home/ PC/CC													
de Silva-Sanigorski, 2010[188]	N	Y	Australia	NR	0-5	NR	NR	43,811	208	NR	[2-4]	NR	NR
Community/ School/ PC/CC													
Chang, 2010[189]	N	Y	JS	NR	NR	NR	NR	NR	208	NR	NR	NR	WNH, Arm1:35.9) Arm2:(35.4) Arm3:(22.9) Arm4:(38) Arm5:(37.3)

API = Asian Pacific Islander; BMI = body mass index (in kg/m^2); BNH = Black non-Hispanic, N = no; NR = not reported; RCT = randomized controlled trials; WNH = White non-Hispanic; Y = yes*Inclusion/exclusion criteria.
[†]Participant characteristics.

Table 33. Interventions of studies based in the community

Author, Year	Control Arm	Description of Intervention	Diet (Phys/Env)	Diet (Psych)	Physical Activity (Phys/Env)	Physical Activity (Psych)
Community Only						
Eiholzer, 2010[182]	Usual care	The resistance exercise program consisted of supervised 1-hour exercise sessions twice weekly.			X	X
Community/ School						
Sallis, 2003[75]	Usual care	School activities/components including physical education classes, school food sources. Statewide regulatory changes to reduce sedentary behavior and promote healthy lifestyle; childcare technical assistance; training around healthy habits.	X		X	X
Singh, 2009[183]	Usual care	Classroom based educational program that covered 11 lessons for the subjects of biology and physical education. Aimed at raising awareness and information processing with regard to energy balance–related behaviors; Aimed at facilitation of choice to improve 1 of the risk behaviors.	X	X	X	X
Chomitz, 2010[184]	Usual care	Healthy eating and active living through a poster campaign, newsletters, mini-grants. Innovative food service projects such as new recipe and menu development and cafeteria taste-tests were developed. Raise community awareness of resources available in the city to promote active living through a poster campaign. Physical education programs were implemented at all 12 K-8 schools similarly to improve access to physical activity opportunities.	X	X	X	X
Community/ School/ Home						
Economos, 2007[185]	Usual care	Breakfast program; walk to school campaign; professional development for staff; school food service; classroom curriculum; Enhanced recess; school wellness policy development; after school SUS curriculum; walk from school campaign. Parent outreach and educational information; family events; nutrition forums; Child's health report card. Community or environment-level: SUS Community Advisory Council; Ethnic-minority collaborations; walking trainings; Farmers Market; City Employee Wellness Campaign; SUS approved restaurants; SUS 5K & Fitness fair; media placement; collaboration on health events.	X	X	X	X

Table 33. Interventions of studies based in the community (continued)

Author, Year	Control Arm	Description of Intervention	Diet (Phys/Env)	Diet (Psych)	Physical Activity (Phys/Env)	Physical Activity (Psych)
Community/ Home						
Klesges, 2012[187]	Both groups received the same intervention for 1 year. After first year program included social awareness and community responsibility	Practical experience with nutrition and physical activity by way of interactive learning. The girls developed behavioral goals to eat a nutritional diet, increase physical activity, and reduce sedentary activity.		X		X
Robinson, 2010[186]	Usual care	Daily 1-hour homework period and small snack followed by 45 to 60 minutes of learning and practicing dance routines. Home-based screen time reduction intervention designed to incorporate African or African American history and culture.	X			X
Community/ Home/ PC/CC						
de Silva-Sanigorski, 2010[188]	Usual care	Increase awareness of key messages in homes, primary care, and childcare settings. Promote healthy eating, distribute water bottles, active play.	X	X	X	X
Community/ School/ PC/CC						
Chang, 2010[189]	Usual care	Wellness programs; assessment of student fitness; promote healthy eating/physical education/activity, training of childcare providers about healthy behaviors. Implementation of Expert Committee recommendations on assessment, prevention and treatment of child and adolescent overweight. Implementation of policy and practice changes with organizations such as YMCA Childcare	X	X	X	X

CC = childcare; PC = primary care; Psych = psychosocial intervention; Phys/Env = physical/environmental intervention

133

Outcomes

Diet Interventions
None reported.

Physical Activity Interventions

Weight-Related Outcomes

Percent Body Fat
There was no difference in percent body fat between the intervention and control groups at baseline and followup (Appendix E, Evidence Table 54a).[182]

Clinical Outcomes
None reported.

Adverse Events
None reported.

Intermediate Outcomes
This study reported a significant increase in physical activity ($p=0.01$) as indicated by in the spontaneous activity energy expenditure (SpAEE), kcal/min (Appendix E, Evidence Table 54b).[182]

Interpretation
The results from an outcome measure from one community only-based study reporting on a physical activity intervention support our conclusion. The study reported on percent body fat and showed no significant change over 1 year. However, it did show a significant increase in physical activity. The study enrolled a small sample of boys only and aimed to increase spontaneous activity. It did not include dietary components. We need more physical activity interventions among larger, more diverse populations to further evaluate the impact of these interventions.

Diet and Physical Activity Interventions
None reported.

Strength of the Evidence

Weight-Related Outcomes
The strength of evidence is insufficient that community-only based physical activity interventions prevent obesity or overweight in children (Table 34; Appendix F, Strength of Evidence Table 1).

Intermediate Outcomes
There was insufficient evidence to grade intermediate outcomes of physical activity interventions.

Table 34. Summary of the strength of evidence for weight-related outcomes in studies taking place in community-only settings

Setting	Intervention, n	Years of Publication	Enrolled Participants	Studies With Low/ Moderate/ High Risk of Bias(n)	% With Favorable (Statistically Sig) Outcome	% With Favorable Outcome (Does Not Need to be Stat Sig)	Risk of Bias	Consistency	Precision	Directness	Strength of the Evidence
Community-only	PA, 1	2010	46	0/1/0	0	0	Moderate	NA	Imprecise	Direct	Insufficient

PA = physical activity intervention; NA = not applicable

135

Community–School–Based Studies

Study Characteristics

There were three studies, including two RCTs,[75,183] and one non-RCT.[184] Their stated goal was obesity prevention or weight maintenance. Two studies took place in the U.S.,[75,184] and the other in the Netherlands.[183] Two studies did not report inclusion criteria,[75,183] the other only included children under 5 years old (Table 32; Appendix E, Evidence Table 55).[184]

Population Characteristics

Two studies included a total of 2,966 participants and one study included 24 schools with a mean enrollment of 1,109 at each school. One study had a followup of 156 weeks,[184], one study had a followup of between 32-80 weeks[183], and one study had a followup of 104 weeks[75] The proportion of females ranged from 48.2[184] to 53.3[183] percent in these studies. Two studies did not report on age.[183] Mean age ranged from 7.7 years[184] to 12.7 years.[183] None of the studies reported on the grade of the participants. Two studies reported on race (Table 32; Appendix E, Evidence Table 56).[75,184]

Interventions

All three studies reported on combined diet and physical activity interventions (Table 33; Appendix E, Evidence Table 57).[183]

Outcomes

Diet Interventions

None Reported.

Physical Activity Interventions

None Reported.

Diet and Physical Activity Interventions

Weight-Related Outcomes

BMI z-Score

One study reported on change in BMI z score and showed a decrease (0.67 vs. 0.63, $p < 0.001$) (Appendix E, Evidence Table 58a,b).[184]

BMI

Two studies reported on BMI. One did not observe any differences in BMI between the intervention and control groups[183] and one observed differences among males but not females[75] (Appendix E, Evidence Table 58a,b).

Prevalence of Overweight and Obesity

One study reported on the prevalence of obesity and showed a decrease (20.2 percent vs. 18.0 percent, $p < 0.05$) (Appendix E, Evidence Table 58a,b).[184]

This study also reported on subgroups; the sum of skinfold thickness was lower in girls in intervention schools at both a 32-week followup (-2.3mm; 95% CI: -4.3, -0.03mm) and 240-week followup (-2.0mm; 95% CI: -3.9, -0.1mm) (Appendix E, Evidence Table 58).[183] Additionally, Black and Hispanic children were more likely to be obese at baseline (27 percent and 28.5 percent, respectively) compared to white (12.6 percent) and Asian children (14.3 percent). But obesity along all race/ethnicity groups declined during the study (Appendix E, Evidence Table 58a,b).

Waist Circumference

One study reported on waist circumference change. For males, waist circumference was lower in the intervention group at a 32-week followup (-0.6cm; 95% CI: -1.1 to -0.1cm), but at a 20-month followup waist circumference was significantly lower in the control group (Appendix E, Evidence Table 58a,b).[183]

Skinfold Thickness

One study reported on skinfold thickness change. At the 240 week followup, bicep skinfold thickness among females was lower (-0.7mm; 95% CI: -1.3, -0.04mm) (Appendix E, Evidence Table 58a,b).[183]

Clinical Outcomes

None reported.

Adverse Events

None reported.

Intermediate Outcomes

Physical Activity and Sedentary Behavior

One study measured the impact of this intervention on endurance and fitness.[184] The percent that passed the endurance cardiovascular test significantly increased from 52.6 to 66.6 percent (14.0 percent increase, $p < 0.001$) in the intervention group. One study[183] measured active commuting (walking) to school and found no significant difference between groups. This study also reported on consumption of sugar-sweetened beverages and found no difference between the control and interventions. One study measured moderate to vigorous physical activity, sedentary hours, and fatty foods and found no significant differences between groups (Appendix E, Evidence Table 58c).

Interpretation

The results from outcome measures from two community/school-based studies reporting on combined interventions support our conclusions. One study reported on BMI z-score and showed a significant decrease. Two studies reported on BMI and one showed a significant decrease. These interventions focused on education and environmental changes promoting a healthy diet and physical activity. We may need more interventions combining diet and physical activity to further evaluate the impact of these interventions.

Strength of the Evidence

Weight-Related Outcomes

The strength of evidence is moderate that community/school based diet and physical activity interventions prevent obesity or overweight in children (Table 35, Appendix F, Strength of Evidence Table 1). No studies measured adverse events.

Intermediate Outcomes

There was insufficient evidence to grade intermediate outcomes of combination interventions.

Table 35. Summary of the strength of evidence for weight-related outcomes in studies taking place in community settings with a school component

Setting	Intervention, n	Years of Publication	Enrolled Participants	Studies With Low/ Moderate /High Risk of Bias(n)	% With Favorable (Statistically Sig) utcome	% With Favorable Outcome (Does Not Need to be Stat Sig)	Risk of Bias	Consistency	Precision	Directness	Strength of the Evidence
Community-School	C, 3	1997-2010	2966 and 24 schools (mean enrollment 1,109)	0/3/0	66	66	Moderate	Consistent	Imprecise	Direct	Moderate

C = combination of diet and physical activity interventions

139

Community-School-Home–Based Studies

Study Characteristics

One non-RCT study took place in this setting and the goal of this study was not weight maintenance. This study took place in the U.S. (Table 32; Appendix E, Evidence Table 59).[185]

Population Characteristics

This study included 1,178 participants whose mean age was between 7.3 and 7.9 years old. Participants were in grades 1-3, and were of mixed ethnicity (Table 32; Appendix E, Evidence Table 60).[185]

Interventions

This study reported on a combination of diet and physical activity intervention (Table 33; Appendix E, Evidence Table 61).[185]

Outcomes

Diet Interventions

None reported.

Physical Activity Interventions

None reported.

Diet and Physical Activity Interventions

One non-RCT reported on a diet, physical activity and change in sedentary behavior intervention.[185] The study randomized 1,178 participants and analyzed 1,178 at 43 weeks.

Weight-Related Outcomes

BMI z-Score

In the intervention community, BMI z-score decreased by -0.1005 ($p = 0.001$) compared with children in the control communities (Appendix E, Evidence Table 62a,b).[185]

Clinical Outcomes

None reported.

Adverse Events

None reported.

Intermediate Outcomes

None reported.

Interpretations

The results from outcome measures from one community/school/home-based study reporting on a combination intervention support our conclusions. This study showed a significant decrease in BMI z-score over 1 year. The study was conducted in a community in Massachusetts with components in the school and the home. We need more diet and physical activity intervention studies among diverse populations.

Strength of the Evidence

Weight-Related Outcomes

The strength of evidence is insufficient that community/school/home based interventions which target a combination of diet and physical activity prevent obesity or overweight in children. No studies measured adverse events. No studies measured intermediate outcomes (Table 36, Appendix F, Strength of Evidence Table 1).

Table 36. Summary of the strength of evidence for weight-related outcomes in studies taking place in community settings with a school and home component

Setting	Intervention, n	Years of Publication	Enrolled Participants	Studies With Low/ Moderate/ High Risk of Bias(n)	% With Favorable (Statistically Sig) Outcome	% With Favorable Outcome (Does Not Need to be Stat Sig)	Risk of Bias	Consistency	Precision	Directness	Strength of the Evidence
Community-School-Home	C, 1	2007-2008	1326	0/1/0	100	100	Moderate	NA	Imprecise	Direct	Insufficient

C = combination of diet and physical activity interventions

Community-Home–Based Studies

Study Characteristics

Two RCTs were included in this setting.[186,187] Both studies included only girls in elementary school who were African-American girls aged 8 to 10 years old.[186,187] One study included only participants with a BMI at or higher than the 25th percentile or had a parent with a BMI of 25 or higher[187] (Table 32; Appendix E, Evidence Table 63).

Population Characteristics

The two studies include 924 participants. Length of followup was 104 weeks for both studies. Participants were on average 9.3 to 9.4 years old and were all African-American (Table 32; Appendix E, Evidence Table 64).[186]

Interventions

Both studies tested a combined diet and physical activity intervention (Table 33; Appendix E, Evidence Table 65).[186,187]

Outcomes

Diet Interventions
None reported.

Physical Activity Interventions
None reported.

Diet and Physical Activity Interventions

Weight-Related Outcomes

BMI z-Score
Changes in BMI z-score did not differ between the two intervention groups (Appendix E, Evidence Table 66a).[186]

BMI
Changes in BMI did not differ between the intervention group and the control for either study (Appendix E, Evidence Table 66a).[186,187]

Prevalence of Overweight and Obesity
Changes in BMI $\geq$ 95th percentile did not differ between the two intervention groups. (Appendix E, Evidence Table 66a).[186]

Waist Circumference
Changes in waist circumference did not differ between the intervention group and the control for either study (Appendix E, Evidence Table 66a).[186,187]

Skinfold Thickness
    Changes in triceps skinfold did not differ between intervention group and the control for either study (Appendix E, Evidence Table 66a).[186,187]

Clinical Outcomes
    Changes in systolic blood pressure did not differ between the two intervention groups. Changes in diastolic blood pressure did not differ between the two intervention groups (Appendix E, Evidence Table 66b).[186]

Adverse Events
    None reported.

Intermediate Outcomes

Physical Activity and Sedentary Behavior
    Group difference in changes in the intermediate outcomes including weekday, weekend and after-school moderate-to-vigorous physical activity, weekday/weekend screen time, total daily energy intake as well as average percentage of energy from fat were all in the expected direction, but did not reach statistical significance (Appendix E, Evidence Table 66c).[186,187]

Physical Activity and Sedentary Behavior
    One study reported on change in dietary intake. This study reported on sugar sweetened beverage intake, and found a nonsignificant decrease in favor of the intervention. This study reported a significant increase in water consumption in the intervention group (p=0.02). Fruit and vegetable intake also increased in the intervention group but was not significant (p=0.07) (Appendix E, Evidence Table 66c).[187]

Interpretation
    We can make limited conclusions regarding community- and home-based studies reporting diet and physical activity interventions. The studies reported on BMI z-score, BMI, waist circumference, and skinfold thickness over two years but did not show significant differences between the two groups. The studies took place among small samples of African-American girls. The health education and physical activity interventions took place in different study groups; therefore the participants did not receive both the diet and physical activity intervention. We need more diet and physical activity intervention studies among larger, more diverse populations to further evaluate the impact of this intervention.

Strength of the Evidence

Weight-Related Outcomes
    The strength of evidence is insufficient that community/ home-based interventions using a combined diet and physical activity intervention prevent obesity or overweight in children (Table 37, Appendix F, Strength of Evidence Table 1).

Intermediate Outcomes
    There was insufficient evidence to grade intermediate outcomes of combined diet and physical activity interventions (Appendix F, Strength of Evidence Tables 2 and 7).

Table 37. Summary of the strength of evidence for weight-related outcomes in studies taking place in community settings with a home component

Setting	Intervention, n	Years of Publication	Enrolled Participants	Studies With Low/ Moderate/ High Risk of Bias(n)	% With Favorable (Statistically Sig) Outcome	% With Favorable Outcome (Does Not Need to be Stat Sig)	Risk of Bias	Consistency	Precision	Directness	Strength of the Evidence
Community-Home	C, 2	2010	564	0/1/1	0	0	Moderate	Consistent	Imprecise	Direct	Insufficient

C = combination diet and physical activity interventions; NA = not applicable

Community-Home-Primary Care and Childcare–Based Studies

Study Characteristics

We included one quasi-experimental Australian study that took place in this setting and had a stated goal of obesity prevention. The study reported on a diet, physical activity, and change in sedentary behavior[188]. The study randomized 2,202 participants and analyzed 2,393 at 103 weeks. This study included children between the ages of 0 and 5 years old. The study did not report any other inclusion criteria (Table 32; Appendix E, Evidence Table 67).[188]

Population Characteristics

This study included a total of 43,811 participants whose mean age was between 2 and 4 years old. The study did not report any other participant characteristics (Table 32; Appendix E, Evidence Table 68).[188]

Interventions

This study investigated the combination intervention of diet and physical activity (Table 33; Appendix E, Evidence Table 69).[188]

Outcomes

Diet Interventions

None reported.

Physical Activity Interventions

None reported.

Diet and Physical Activity Interventions

Weight-Related Outcomes

BMI z-Score

In the intervention group, there was a significantly lower BMI z-score in the 3.5-year-old subsample (0.67 vs. 0.54, $p < 0.05$) (Appendix E, Evidence Table 70a,b).[188]

BMI

In the intervention group, there was a significantly lower BMI in the 3.5-year-old subsample (16.35 kg/m^2 vs. 16.17 kg/m^2, $p < 0.05$) (Appendix E, Evidence Table 70a,b).[188]

Weight

In the intervention group, there was a significantly lower weight in the 3.5-year-old subsample (17.05 kg vs. 16.76 kg, $p < 0.05$) (Appendix E, Evidence Table 70a,b).[188]

Prevalence of Overweight and Obesity

In the intervention group, there was a significantly lower prevalence of overweight/obesity in the 2 and 3.5-year-old subsample (by 2.5 and 3.4 percentage points, respectively) than there was in the comparison sample (a difference of 0.7 percentage points, p < 0.05) (Appendix E, Evidence Table 70a,b).[188]

Clinical Outcomes
None reported.

Adverse Events
None reported.

Intermediate Outcomes
None reported.

Interpretation
We can make no conclusions regarding community, home, primary care, and childcare-based studies reporting on a combined intervention. The single study showed a significant decrease in BMI, BMI z-score, and weight among young children (3.5 years) over 4 years. The study took place in a community in Australia with components in the school, primary care, and child-care settings. We need more diet and physical activity interventions among diverse populations to further evaluate the impact of this intervention.

Strength of the Evidence
The strength of evidence is insufficient that community-home-primary care-child-care -based diet and physical activity interventions prevent obesity or overweight in children (Table 38, Appendix F, Strength of Evidence Table 1).

Table 38. Summary of the strength of evidence for weight-related outcomes in studies taking place in community settings with home, primary care, and child-care components

Setting	Intervention, n	Years of Publication	Enrolled Participants	Studies With Low/ Moderate/ High Risk of Bias(n)	% With Favorable (Statistically Sig) Outcome	% With Favorable Outcome (Does Not Need to be Stat Sig)	Risk of Bias	Consistency	Precision	Directness	Strength of the Evidence
Community -Home-PC- CC	C, 1	2010	43,811	0/1/0	100	100	Moderate	NA	Imprecise	Direct	Insufficient

C = combination diet and physical activity interventions; NA = not applicable; PC=primary care; CC = childcare

148

Community-School-Primary Care-Childcare–Based Studies

Study Characteristics

We included one quasi-experimental study conducted in the U.S. in this setting with the stated goal of obesity prevention. The study reported on a combined diet and physical activity intervention, which randomized 2,202 participants[189]. It did not define any inclusion criteria (Table 32; Appendix E, Evidence Table 71).[189]

Population Characteristics

This study included a total of 2,202 participants. It did not report any other participant characteristics (Table 32; Appendix E, Evidence Table 72).[189]

Interventions

This study investigated a diet intervention (Table 33; Appendix E, Evidence Table 73).[189]

Outcomes

Diet Interventions

None reported

Physical Activity Interventions

None reported.

Diet and Physical Activity Interventions

Weight-Related Outcomes

Prevalence of Overweight and Obesity

In the intervention group, there was no significant change in the prevalence of obesity (20.6 vs. 24.2 percent) or prevalence of overweight (17 vs. 17 percent) (Appendix E, Evidence Table 74a).[189]

Clinical Outcomes

None reported.

Adverse Events

None reported.

Intermediate Outcomes

None reported.

Interpretation

We can make no conclusions regarding community, school, primary care, and child-care center-based studies reporting on a combined intervention. The single diet and physical activity study showed no significant change in the prevalence of obesity over three years. The study took place in a community in Delaware with components in the school, primary care and child-care settings. We need more diet and physical activity interventions among diverse populations to further evaluate the impact of these interventions.

Strength of the Evidence

Weight-Related Outcomes

The strength of evidence is insufficient that community/ home/primary care/child-care center-based combined diet and physical activity interventions prevent obesity or overweight in children (Table 39, Appendix F, Strength of Evidence Table 1). No studies measured adverse events.

Table 39. Summary of the strength of evidence for weight-related outcomes in studies taking place in community settings with school, primary care, and child-care components

Setting	Intervention, n	Years of Publication	Enrolled Participants	Studies With Low/ Moderate/ High Risk of Bias(n)	% With favorable (Statistically Sig) Outcome	% With Favorable Outcome (Does Not Need to be Stat Sig)	Risk of Bias	Consistency	Precision	Directness	Strength of the Evidence
Community-School-PC-CC	C, 1	2010	NR	0/0/1	100	100	High	Inconsistent	Imprecise	Direct	Insufficient

C = combination diet and physical activity intervention; NA = not applicable; PC = primary care; CC = childcare

151

Key Question 6: What is the comparative effectiveness of consumer health informatics applications for the prevention of obesity or overweight in children?

We identified six studies that met our inclusion criteria that evaluated the effects of consumer health informatics (CHI) interventions, but they took place primarily in other settings, and thus we reported them under other KQs.

KQ 1 included five studies with a consumer health informatics component: four on school-based setting with a CHI component to the intervention,[165-168] and one on school-based setting with a home and CHI component.[170] Two of the school-CHI studies reported on physical activity interventions and showed no significant intervention effect on weight outcomes,[165,167] and two reported on combined diet and physical activity interventions,[166,168] and one showed a significant intervention effect on BMI (p<0.001),[166] while the other failed to show an intervention effect. The study reporting on the school-home-CHI intervention used a combined diet and physical activity intervention and demonstrated no intervention effect on weight outcomes.[170]

KQ 2 included one study with a CHI component: the study took place in a home-based setting with primary care and CHI components.[175] This study used a combination diet and physical activity intervention and showed no difference in BMI z-score between the intervention and control during followup after adjusting for baseline BMI z-score, age, and ethnicity, and significant improvements in sedentary behaviors for both genders and active days per week among boys. Subgroup analysis for participants with BMI at or above 95th percentile showed a desirable but insignificant intervention effect: BMI z-score was 2.08±0.02 for intervention and 2.12±0.02 for the control during followup (P=.10).The intervention did not demonstrate an overall effect on BMI z scores.

The six CHI intervention studies identified only took place in concert with other interventions, primarily school-based, and also home-based physical activity and dietary interventions. CHI interventions contributed to improvements in intermediate outcomes, particularly physical activity, but only one[166] of these six studies, which used a school-based diet and physical activity intervention, in concert with a CHI component, demonstrated a change in weight outcomes.

Discussion

Key Findings

We identified 124 interventional studies (described in 131 articles) meeting our inclusion criteria, of which 54 took place in the United States and 70 were in other developed countries. Eighty-three studies were RCTs. The majority (104 studies, 84 percent) were school-based studies, although many of them also included interventions implemented in other settings such as in the home or local community. Few studies tested interventions that were primarily implemented in other settings such as at home, in communities, in primary care settings, or in childcare settings.

The evidence is strong to support some interventions. The school based studies of physical activity, which included a home component, all improved obesity outcomes. Two of the three studies targeted a reduction in sedentary activity which may have contributed to the good outcomes. Combination interventions of diet and physical activity interventions in schools, with home and community components, also effectively improved outcomes (Table 40).

Additionally, there is moderate evidence that using dietary interventions or physical activity interventions, alone, in schools prevent obesity. The dietary interventions in the school setting included education of the children which may have contributed to their success. However, the paucity of studies makes it hard to know why these particular interventions worked. The strength of the evidence is also moderate that combinations of diet and physical activity in school, with a home component, positively impacts obesity prevalence. The diet and physical activity interventions included enhanced classroom physical activity lessons, moderate to vigorous physical activity sessions, nutritional education materials, and healthful diet promotion (Table 40).

The strength of evidence is low that diet and physical activity interventions administered at home, or in child-care facilities, prevent obesity or overweight in children. Those interventions with significant parental or family involvement were able to demonstrate some impact on select intermediate outcomes. However, additional studies with larger sample sizes, greater intensity interventions and longer followup may be necessary to know the impact of diet and physical activity interventions delivered at home. The small sample size and poor quality of the child-care based studies may have contributed to the attenuated effect on weight outcomes (Table 40).

The evidence is insufficient regarding interventions in other settings. This is due primarily to the small number of studies, their moderate or high risk of bias, or conflicting results across studies. We note that there were many studies that combined diet and physical activity interventions in schools and yet the evidence remains insufficient about these combined interventions. These thirty-seven studies had results that were imprecise and largely inconsistent with each other preventing conclusions (Table 40).

Almost all of those studies that reported on intermediate outcomes, such as vegetable and fruit consumption and/or physical activity, detected some statistically significant desirable effects. Similarly, roughly half of the studies that reported clinical outcomes detected some statistically significant desirable effects, predominately lowered blood pressure.

In general, we found that studies done in schools that had large sample sizes, longer follow up, with more vigorous and higher intensity interventions, were more likely to be effective. Comprehensive interventions that promoted environmental changes (e.g., modified food and beverage items offered in school cafeteria, or structural changes in school physical activity) as well as changes in individuals' knowledge and attitude were more likely to be successful than

153

those addressing either one alone. Educational interventions were less likely to be effective than environmental changes. Given that children are exposed to many other influences outside of school, it is heartening to see that interventions implemented in schools can have a significant impact on weight and other outcomes.

Table 40. Summary of conclusions

KQ/Setting	Intervention	Conclusion	SOE
School	Diet	Benefit	Moderate
	Physical activity	Benefit	Moderate
	Combination	No conclusion, inconsistent results	Insufficient
School-Home	Diet	Not enough evidence to reach conclusion	Insufficient
	Physical activity	Benefit	High
	Combination	Benefit	Moderate
School-Home-Community	Physical activity	Not enough evidence to reach conclusion	Insufficient
	Combination	Benefit	High
School-Community	Diet	Not enough evidence to reach conclusion	Insufficient
	Physical activity	Not enough evidence to reach conclusion	Insufficient
	Combination	Benefit	Moderate
School-CHI	Physical activity	No conclusion, inconsistent results	Insufficient
	Combination	No conclusion, inconsistent results	Insufficient
School-Home-CHI	Combination	Not enough evidence to reach conclusion	Insufficient
Home	Diet	Not enough evidence to reach conclusion	Insufficient
	Combination	No benefit	Low
Home-School-Community	Combination	Not enough evidence to reach conclusion	Insufficient
Home-PC-CHI	Combination	Not enough evidence to reach conclusion	Insufficient
Primary care	Combination	Not enough evidence to reach conclusion	Insufficient
Childcare	Combination	No benefit	Low
	Physical activity	Not enough evidence to reach conclusion	Insufficient
Community	Physical activity	Not enough evidence to reach conclusion	Insufficient
Community-school	Combination	Benefit	Moderate
Community-School-Home	Combination	Not enough evidence to reach conclusion	Insufficient
Community-Home	Combination	No conclusion, high risk of bias studies	Insufficient
Community-Home-PC-CC	Combination	Not enough evidence to reach conclusion	Insufficient
Community-Home-PC-CC	Combination	Not enough evidence to reach conclusion	Insufficient

Combination = combination of a diet and physical activity intervention; CHI = consumer thelath informatics; CC = childcare; PC = primary care

Important Unanswered Questions

What Is the Optimal Setting for Childhood Obesity Prevention Interventions?

This review did not aim to compare interventions across settings, and it remains an unanswered question as to where interventions are best implemented. Are physical activity interventions most effective when implemented in school or in an aftercare setting? Is diet education most effective when done in school or at home visits?

This review confirmed that most obesity prevention interventions have been tested in schools, consistent with previous findings.[190,191] An Institute of Medicine report on childhood obesity recommended school as the national focal point for obesity prevention in the U.S.[192] We suggest, however, that while the school is the setting most commonly studied, it may not be the optimal setting for obesity prevention programs. Many experts support that obesity is driven by a host of environmental factors which increase opportunities for energy intake and decrease opportunities for energy expenditure.[193] Obesity-prevention interventions based in schools may not be effective in reducing the risks posted in other settings. When sufficient studies have been conducted, cross-setting analysis of interventions will be desirable. Head-to-head comparisons of comparable interventions delivered in disparate settings may be needed.

What Are the Other Beneficial Effects and Unwanted Consequences of Obesity Prevention?

We hypothesized that obesity prevention programs could result in desirable clinical outcomes even when the intervention did not result in weight control. In this report, we describe select clinical outcomes that are influenced by obesity, including blood pressure and blood lipids and the effect of interventions. The question is whether interventions that affect only intermediate outcomes, like dietary choices and physical activity, also have a beneficial effect on health. Given the long interval between exposure and the outcomes, these hypotheses are difficult to test and typically require observational designs.

Obesity prevention interventions may also result in some unwanted consequences for children and their families, such as stigma,[194] low self-esteem,[195] injury (due to physical activity), eating disorders,[196] or impaired growth.[197] However, very few studies we reviewed reported on such adverse effects. Failure to report adverse effects can mask the reasons for why the interventions generally showed small effects. Low self-esteem or stigmatization as a result of the intervention may reduce fidelity to the intervention and hinder participants from adhering.

Does the Effectiveness of Obesity Prevention Differ in Subgroups?

A few studies examined whether the effect of the intervention varied across groups defined by gender, age, or baseline weight status, but reported mixed results. Very few studies examined other characteristics, such as race/ethnicity or socio-economic status. We need future research focusing on sub-populations. In some studies, children with different socio-demographic characteristics responded differently to the same intervention. For example, a combined dietary and physical activity intervention that involved the children's schools, homes, and communities was effective in elementary school children, but not in middle-school students.[148] Another intervention provided health and nutrition education to pupils in Crete and found girls to be more responsive to the intervention than boys.[78] A community-based after-school program found an important decrease in BMI z-scores among Asian American children, with an unanticipated increase in African American children.[162] Such differences may be explained by fidelity to the intervention, cultural responses to the intervention, or differences in growth patterns. However, evidence is still limited to explain this variation.

Our limited findings related to sub-populations are similar to previous reviews. For example, one review reported that efforts to prevent weight gain were more effective in children aged 6 to 12 than in older children.[191] Another review found that girls may be more responsive to interventions built on the social learning theory, while boys may be more responsive to structural or environmental approaches.[198] This suggests the need for stratified analyses of pre-specified sub-groups to assess the effects of the interventions in these subgroups.

Findings in Relationship to What Is Already Known

In general, our main findings are consistent with previous systematic reviews. However, we are unaware of other reviews which have provided a comprehensive examination of diverse study settings like ours. Most other reviewers mainly focused on select settings such as school and on select outcomes such as BMI or prevalence of overweight and obesity. This review also provides some new findings. We found that a large majority (103, 82 percent) of the 125 studies are school-based, and few studies have tested interventions in other settings. Previous reviews[190,198,199] have focused primarily on schools, while a few recent reviews examined other settings.[191,200] Earlier reviews focused primarily on weight outcomes, such as BMI, while we included various weight and adiposity outcomes as well as clinical and intermediate outcomes. We also described adverse effects.

The results of previous reviews looking at the impact obesity prevention on weight outcomes in the school setting are mixed. Some did not detect significant intervention effects, while some did.[191,200] Most reviews described modest or mixed effects of obesity prevention interventions in children across all settings,[201-203] or within schools;[190,198] and there was limited evidence in support of school policies and regulations.[199] The inconsistent findings are largely due to differences in the design of the reviews, their methods, and the quality of the primary literature (e.g., small study size, lack of blinding, short followup, and varied statistical analyses.[191,203,204]

Overall, our findings are consistent with the Institute of Medicine's recommendations [192] about obesity prevention. The Institute of Medicine reported that a) the school is the most frequent setting to be studied and included in meta-analysis or review; b) despite small effect sizes and sometimes inconsistent evidence, there is a cumulative body of research showing that school-based interventions can prevent obesity; c) school-based interventions modifying both diet and physical activity are more effective in preventing childhood obesity than modifying either diet or physical activity alone; d) school-based interventions, with family or community involvement, are more likely to be effective; e) different stakeholders, including governments, community, health care systems, industry, and educators should work together to modify the obesogenic environment to facilitate healthful behaviors;[205]and f) we need more research to test interventions in settings other than schools, in particular, those that test environmental and policy changes, as well as those in clinical settings.

However, discrepancies between findings from our study and previous reviews still exist, especially in the magnitude of intervention effect. For example, while our study generally found a low to moderate intervention effect for school-based intervention programs (with a few exceptions of large intervention effect for physical activity interventions in school-home settings and combined diet and physical activity interventions in school-community settings), the most recent Cochrane review on childhood obesity preventions showed strong evidence to support the beneficial effects of school-based intervention programs for children, particularly among those aged 6 to12 years,[205] while another systematic review on 18 studies did not find any significant improvements in BMI from school-based physical activity interventions.[206]

Applicability

The results of this review are primarily applicable to children in high-income countries. Results are not necessarily applicable to children in middle-and low-income countries. The children enrolled in the reviewed studies were diverse across studies, with a mix of girls and boys of multiple ethnic groups. However, only a small number of studies reported outcomes by the subgroups of sex, race/ethnicity, or age. Therefore, one should apply the results cautiously to subgroups of children, particularly subgroups that only a few studies included, such as very young children and select racial/ethnic groups. Also, prevention strategies that were effective in old studies may not be as effective in current populations due to differences in the social and build environments.

We gave more weight in our evidence grading to RCTs than non-RCTs). For the most part, the RCTs included in this review took place in school settings. Thus, there may be a relative understating of the value of interventions in non-school settings.

Implications for Clinical and Policy Decisionmaking

The findings from this review can help guide decision making by researchers, clinicians, public health practitioners, and policymakers about the most effective settings and types of interventions for preventing childhood obesity in developed countries. Based on these results and the results of previous reviews, school-based interventions are likely to remain a focal point for prevention interventions. The limited number of studies conducted outside school limits the evidence about the effectiveness of interventions in those settings.

We anticipate that the school will remain a key setting for health promotion, including for childhood obesity prevention. Several factors favor school-focused efforts: (1) it is easier to conduct continuous interventions and followup measurements in school than in less standardized settings; (2) dietary and exercise behaviors at school constitute a large proportion of children's daily diet and physical activity; (3) schools have the relevant infrastructure to deliver intervention and evaluation, including annual physical check-ups, nutrition and physical education teachers, and school nurses; (4) the majority of school-age children in high-income countries attend and spend considerable time at school; and (5) the evidence supports the effectiveness of some school-based interventions.

To date, it has been unclear whether physical activity or diet (or the combination) should be the primary focus of population-based obesity intervention programs. We found a higher strength of evidence for physical activity interventions in schools that included a home component than for diet-only interventions. However, studies testing these interventions head-to-head were rare, so our review does not definitely answer this question. Nevertheless, to maintain a desirable energy balance, it may be easier to control energy intake than to increase energy expenditure, as there are biological limitations to the effectiveness of physical activity alone in controlling body weight, as well as social and environmental challenges to fitting activity into children's daily schedule. In addition, the environmental factors that affect food consumption in schools might be easier and less costly to modify than those affecting physical activity. However, we note that there may be opportunity costs if schools are required to divert attention and resources to these activities at the expense of other learning or enrichment activities.

Policy change is difficult to effect; nevertheless, in recent years, there is strong interest in the U.S. and some other industrialized countries to push community and policy based interventions. It is likely that with the growing government and public support, such interventions could become more feasible and sustainable in the future. We note that although the evidence is insufficient to address harms, policy makers implementing intervention programs might consider *potential* harms, which may include self-esteem effects, a sense of failure, and time diverted from other activities. When choosing an intervention to implement, decision makers need to consider the availability of resources; the costs, potential harms and unwanted consequences of an intervention; the anticipated magnitude of the effectiveness of the program, as well as the other underlying issues contributing to the obesity problem specific to their population, such as specific risk factors and other competitive needs.

Limitations of the Evidence Review Process

This review included only studies of normal children in high-income countries, thereby limiting the generalizability of these findings to high-risk groups and low- and middle-income countries.

Publication bias is inevitable in this review, as journals are less likely to publish intervention studies failing to achieve a desirable effect. We partially addressed this bias, as we searched for "gray literature" (e.g. unpublished working papers) to include in our review. However, none of the grey literature studies met our inclusion criteria in this search.

Within each study setting, we grouped interventions by their behavioral changes (e.g., diet, physical activity, or both) although the studies might have applied very different intervention approaches. However, due to the limited number of studies by categories, we could not conduct further stratifications and analyses to explore the comparative effectiveness of the specific intervention approaches (e.g., education intervention vs. environmental change), or specific intermediate outcomes (e.g., fruits and vegetable intake vs. total energy intake). Moreover, none of the interventions was identical to another. We synthesized the evidence at the level of the intervention – this may be interpreted as "physical activity" is beneficial or as "both diet and PA" is beneficial – even if the report cannot support what specific intervention has the strongest evidence relative to another.

For studies with multiple time points during followup assessments, we mainly included the final one, reasoning that the final followup could best demonstrate how the effect of a specific intervention sustains over time. Including multiple time points for one study would inflate the influence of the study when summarizing the evidence; this may also cause problems as the length of different interventions in one setting may vary greatly based on the final followup lengths.

For school-based studies, we reduced the requirement for length of followup to 6 months (from 1 year) considering the usual length of school years. However, 6 months may be short to observe an intervention's effect on weight outcomes. It may be desirable to conduct in depth analysis to compare the findings from small, short-term (e.g., 6 months) studies with those form large, well-designed RCTs. However, we are limited by the scope of this review, the large heterogeneity across studies and small number of comparable studies. Some studies did not report the original study goals and some studies did not target obesity, that is, they targeted cardiovascular risks. These studies were included in this review because they had diet and physical activity interventions and reported body weight-related outcomes. Since these studies might differ from those that target childhood obesity prevention, they add heterogeneity to the study pool and yet provide valuable information on childhood obesity prevention.

We attempted to identify studies reported in languages other than English, but none of those met our inclusion criteria. As a result, one should exercise caution when generalizing findings from this review to non-English speaking populations.

Limitations of the Evidence Base

There are also limitations with the evidence base. There are many differences across studies in term of countries, settings (e.g., school vs. home), design (e.g., RCTs versus non-RCTs), sample size, sample characteristics (e.g., all white versus mixed race/ethnicity), specific intervention approaches (e.g., nutrition seminars vs. change in school café menus), primary measures that assess intervention effects (e.g., BMI vs. prevalence of obesity), length of followup, and statistical analysis approaches (e.g. F-tests vs. multi-level models). Such variability made it difficult to conduct meta-analyses for most of the various intervention studies we examined. As a result, we could only conduct meta-analysis for select outcomes (mainly BMI or BMI Z score) for KQ 1, and included only a small number of intervention studies in our pooled results.

Moreover, the preponderance of studies conducted in the school setting limits the generalizability of these results to other settings, especially for primary care and childcare.

Few studies reported standard errors or confidence intervals for the weight-related outcomes. In our analysis, we graded studies that did not report measures of variability as imprecise for the body of evidence. In some instances, the studies did not report a mean difference or point estimate and just stated that there was no significant difference in weight change between the groups. This led us to grade the strength of evidence insufficient or low and prevented us from quantitatively pooling results.

Except for the school-based interventions, the strength of evidence was generally low or insufficient for the interventions in other settings. These grades were a result of how we assessed the study quality and strength of evidence (detailed in the methods section). Common reasons for low or insufficient rates were inconsistent findings, a limited number of studies, the lack of blinding, and not accounting for losses to followup.

Since obesity interventions focus on lifestyle modifications, it is difficult to effectively blind participants from knowing whether they are in the intervention or control group. Therefore, we considered blinding to be most essential at the point of group assignment to minimize selection bias, rather than requiring blinding to sustain throughout the intervention phase. This is a reasonable modification and more applicable to this review, but it does allow for reporting bias. For example, participants in the intervention groups who failed to maintain weight and were aware of their group assignment might have refused re-examination, which would result in differential drop-out. The studies we reviewed usually did not report this. Few of the studies reported blinding of outcome assessors, which was likely difficult to implement in these studies.

The measurement of some outcomes, such as physical activity is controversial. There are no consistent standards on how to measure physical activity, especially spontaneous activity. To address this challenge, we formed an ordered list of physical activities, with input from other experts, to guide us in grading the strength of evidence. We made similar lists for weight and other diet-related outcomes.

Weight-related outcomes and statistical methods studies used to evaluate intervention effects were also heterogonous. We used BMI, or related measures such as BMI z-score, BMI percentile, and prevalence of overweight and/or obesity based on BMI cut points as the primary outcome measures. However, BMI is an indirect measure of adiposity and thus has its limitations; it is also not an ideal indicator for cardiometabolic risks. In addition, studies used different BMI cut points to define overweight and obesity. Further, some studies did not even report BMI, making cross-study comparisons difficult.

Lack of reporting some important information, such as process evaluation and program costs, program adherence/fidelity, and adaptations to the local context hinder our exploration in understanding the program effects.

Future Research Needs

Many questions remain unanswered. We have identified a number of evidence gaps, many of which may warrant future research. Many of these are also supported by other reviews.[192,207]

1. Intervention Studies Conducted in Nonschool Settings

The literature is sparse in interventions that take place in settings other than schools. This is identified by our review as well as by others.[192,207] The field needs more studies that test environment- and policy-based interventions. Although environment is a critical area for obesity prevention,[192] very few studies have tested such interventions.[207] In addition, there is scant evidence on the impact of regional or national policies on childhood obesity prevention, including agriculture policies and regulations on food retailing and distributions.[192,207]

Very few studies took place in clinical settings such as primary care. Primary health care providers could play an important role in childhood obesity prevention and treatment by providing healthful eating and exercise guidelines, and regularly monitoring body weight.

2. Innovative Study Design and Intervention Approaches

Innovative interventions could help better target levers for behavioral changes. For example, increasingly, young people in the U.S. and worldwide are using social media, and thus it may be effective to use these modalities to reach these children and adolescents. Using well-developed behavioral theories when designing interventions will help researchers increase study success. For example, only a few studies used social marketing to deliver messages on nutrition, physical activity, and health. Studies can integrate this approach with other intervention components to promote desirable lifestyle changes. Consumer health informatics such as internet and smart phones provide promise for health promotion programs like obesity prevention. However, only six studies used consumer health informatics and only one reported significantly reduced obesity risk.

3. Systems Science Guided Intervention Studies

Obesity in children is the result of a complex mix of biological, behavioral, social, economic, and environmental factors. Thus, the effective and sustainable prevention of obesity in children may have to target many factors, which calls for a systems approach in study design, implementation, and evaluation, that take into account multiple risk factors and the complex interactions and feedback loops among them.[208] To fill in the gaps, researchers first need to understand the contexts and challenges associated with implementing prevention programs in different settings. For example, to conduct a childhood obesity prevention program in a community setting, researchers often need to work with the local community and its key stakeholders, which requires considerable effort and resources. Such demand may help explain the small number of intervention studies conducted in nonschool settings. Researchers should report these contextual factors to help decisionmakers get a better idea of the applicability of a specific intervention program to their own community.

4. Studies That Test Potential Differential Effect of Interventions

We need research that generates information about important sub-groups, such as populations stratified by gender, age, race/ethnicity, or socio-economic status, to test whether different groups may respond differently to the same intervention, and help tailor future interventions to maximize their benefits. To allow for such analysis we may need larger studies, which will be more costly. However, they are essential to provide valuable information for disseminating successful interventions. Such studies will test how different groups may respond to the same intervention differently, and can help tailor future interventions to maximize their benefits. Information about subgroups may lead to interventions that are better targeted, and could thus lead to a more efficient use of resources and better outcomes.

Most of the studies we reviewed did not report results by population subgroup. Subgroup analysis is necessary, as the effect size of a specific intervention may be small due to the heterogeneity of intervention effects among different subgroups. For example, an intervention may have worked in girls but not in boys. This may result in overall effectiveness being insignificant. Future research should include stratified analyses of sub-groups by gender, age, race/ethnicity, or socio-economic status. This will help test how different groups may respond to the same intervention, and help tailor future interventions to maximize their benefits. In addition, studies have found that obesity in older children is more predictive of obesity during adulthood than obesity in younger children.[32] We need more studies to find effective prevention strategies for obesity that occurs in late childhood and adolescence.

5. Studies With High Statistical Power

We need more studies with large sample sizes and adequate length of followup, because most childhood obesity intervention programs are not intensive enough and only result in modest behavioral changes. This is also due to the fact that many factors can affect individuals' eating and physical activity.

6. Publication of Process Evaluation Results on Interventions

The publication of process evaluations should be encouraged, especially those that attempt to compare multiple interventions. Such knowledge is important for translational research and dissemination. Very few of the studies we reviewed reported process evaluation, which would provide useful insights regarding why some studies might detect a desirable effect of the intervention, while others do not.

7. Application of Rigorous Analytic Approaches

We need more rigorous analytic approaches to better analyze the repeated measures collected during the followup, to control for confounders remaining after randomization, and to test effect modification and heterogeneity in the treatment effect.

8. Obesity Prevention Research on Adolescents

Obesity in adolescents has been found to be more predictive of obesity during adulthood than obesity in younger children.[32] We need more studies to find effective prevention strategies for obesity that occurs in late childhood and adolescence. This is an important stage of life when

161

young people are exposed to various social and environmental factors that establish lifelong life habits.

Conclusions

A large number of childhood obesity intervention studies have taken place in high-income counties over the past three decades. They predominately occurred in school settings and mostly in the U.S. Many of the school-based studies also included intervention components implemented in other settings, such as the home and community. Overall, there is moderate-to-high strength of evidence to support that diet and/or physical activity interventions that are implemented in schools help prevent excessive weight gain or reduce the prevalence of overweight and obesity. The added value of school-based interventions, including involvements at home or in the community or the implementation of policies directed at the environment to improve dietary intake or increase physical activity, is generally positive. However, the effectiveness of interventions primarily implemented at home, in primary care, and child-care settings or those using consumer health informatics approaches is largely unknown. We need more research to test interventions conducted in settings other than schools, and to test the impact of policy changes and environmental changes. We should encourage research that tests innovative interventions taking advantage of new technologies, research theories, and methodologies (including systems science). Future research also needs to examine which types of interventions may be more effective and sustainable, and whether subgroups might respond to the same intervention differently.

References

1. Centers for Disease Control (CDC), Childhood Overweight and Obesity, Updated March 31, 2010. www.cdc.gov/obesity/childhood/index.html.

2. Wang Y, Lim H. The global childhood obesity epidemic and the association between socio-economic status and childhood obesity. Int Rev Psychiatry. 2012 June;24(3):176-88. PMID:22724639.

3. Wang Y, Beydoun MA. The obesity epidemic in the United States--gender, age, socioeconomic, racial/ethnic, and geographic characteristics: a systematic review and meta-regression analysis. Epidemiol Rev. 2007; 29:6-28.PMID: 17510091

4. Wang Y, Lobstein T. Worldwide trends in childhood overweight and obesity. Int J Pediatr Obes. 2006;1(1):11-25. PMID: 17902211.

5. Wang Y, Mi J, Shan XY, et al. Is China facing an obesity epidemic and the consequences? The trends in obesity and chronic disease in China. Int J Obes (Lond). 2007 Jan;31(1):177-88. PMID: 16652128.

6. Ogden C, Carroll M, Kit B, et al. Prevalence of obesity and trends in body mass index among US children and adolescents, 1999-2010. JAMA: Journal of the American Medical Association. 2012; 307(5):483-90. PMID: 22253364.

7. Ogden CL, Carroll MD, Flegal KM. High body mass index for age among US children and adolescents, 2003-2006. JAMA. 2008; 299(20):2401-5. PMID: 18505949

8. Birch LL, Anzman-Frasca S. Promoting children's healthy eating in obesogenic environments: Lessons learned from the rat. Physiol Behav. 2011. PMID: 21620880

9. Centers for Disease Control (CDC), 2010b, Overweight & Obesity: Obesity Prevalence Among Low-Income, Preschool-Aged Children 1998-2008, Updated March 16, 2010. www.cdc.gov/obesity/childhood/lowincome.html.

10. Centers for Disease Control (CDC), 2010b, Overweight & Obesity: Obesity Prevalence Among Low-Income, Preschool-Aged Children 1998-2008, Updated March 16, 2010. www.cdc.gov/obesity/childhood/lowincome.html.

11. Ozden MG, Tekin NS, Gurer MA et al. Environmental risk factors in pediatric psoriasis: a multicenter case-control study. Pediatr Dermatol 2011; 28(3):306-12. PMID: 21615473

12. Wang Y, Zhang Q. Are American children and adolescents of low socioeconomic status at increased risk of obesity? Changes in the association between overweight and family income between 1971 and 2002. Am J Clin Nutr. 2006; 84(4):707-16. PMID: 17023695

13. Sallis, J.F., Owen, N. Ecological Models. In: Health Behavior adn Health Education (Theory, Research, and Practice). Glanz K, Lewis FM, Nad Rimer K., Eds. 2nd Ed. Jossey-Bass. San Francisco. 1997: 403-424.

14. World Health Organization. Global Strategy on Diet, Physical Activity, and Health. www.who.int/dietphysicalactivity/childhood_what_can_be_done/en/index.html.

15. Institute of Medicine. Preventing Childhood Obesity: Health in the Balance. 2005 www.nap.edu/catalog.php?record_id=11015.

16. Koplan JP, Liverman CT, Kraak VI. Preventing childhood obesity: health in the balance: executive summary. J Am Diet Assoc. 2005; 105(1):131-8. PMID: 15635359

17. Shiwaku K, Anuurad E, Enkhmaa B, Kitajima K, Yamane Y. Appropriate BMI tor Asian populations. Lancet. 2004; 363(9414):1077. PMID: 15051297

18. Wang Y, Moreno LA, Caballero B, Cole TJ. Limitations of the current world health organization growth references for children and adolescents. Food Nutr Bull. 2006; 27(4 Suppl Growth Standard):S175-88. PMID: 17361655

19. Wang Y. Epidemiology of childhood obesity - Methodological aspects and guidelines: What is new? Int J Obes. 2004; 28(SUPPL. 3):S21-S28. PMID: 15543215

20. Wang Y, Moreno LA, Caballero B, Cole TJ. Limitations of the current world health organization growth references for children and adolescents. Food Nutr Bull 2006; 27(4 Suppl Growth Standard):S175-88. PMID: 17361655

21. Wejdmark AK, Bonnett B, Hedhammar A, Fall T. Lifestyle risk factors for progesterone-related diabetes mellitus in elkhounds - a case-control study. J Small Anim Pract 2011; 52(5):240-5. PMID: 21539568

22. Must A, Dallal GE, Dietz WH. Reference data for obesity: 85th and 95th percentiles of body mass index (wt/ht2) and triceps skinfold thickness. Am J Clin Nutr 1991; 53(4):839-46. PMID: 2008861

23. Kuczmarski RJ, Ogden CL, Grummer-Strawn LM et al. CDC growth charts: United States. Adv Data 2000; (314):1-27. PMID: 11183293

24. Must A, Dallal GE, Dietz WH. Reference data for obesity: 85th and 95th percentiles of body mass index (wt/ht2) and triceps skinfold thickness. Am J Clin Nutr 1991; 53(4):839-46. PMID: 2008861

25. Curatola G, Bolignano D, Rastelli S et al. Ultrafiltration intensification in hemodialysis patients improves hypertension but increases AV fistula complications and cardiovascular events. J Nephrol 2011; 24(4):465-73. PMID: 21534239

26. Mei Z, Grummer-Strawn LM, Pietrobelli A, et al. Validity of body mass index compared with other body-composition screening indexes for the assessment of body fatness in children and adolescents. Am. J. Clin. Nutr. 2002; 75(6):978-85. PMID: 12036802.

27. Pietrobelli A, Faith MS, Allison DB, Gallagher D, Chiumello G, Heymsfield SB. Body mass index as a measure of adiposity among children and adolescents: a validation study. J Pediatr 1998; 132(2):204-10. PMID: 9506629

28. Serdula MK, Ivery D, Coates RJ, Freedman DS, Williamson DF, Byers T. Do obese children become obese adults? A review of the literature. Prev Med 1993; 22(2):167-77. PMID: 8483856

29. Whitaker RC, Wright JA, Pepe MS, Seidel KD, Dietz WH. Predicting obesity in young adulthood from childhood and parental obesity. N Engl J Med 1997; 337(13):869-73. PMID: 9302300

30. Freedman DS, Khan LK, Serdula MK, Dietz WH, Srinivasan SR, Berenson GS. The relation of childhood BMI to adult adiposity: The Bogalusa heart study. Pediatrics. 2005; 115(1):22-7. PMID: 15629977.

31. Freedman DS, Mei Z, Srinivasan SR, Berenson GS, Dietz WH. Cardiovascular risk factors and excess adiposity among overweight children and adolescents: the Bogalusa Heart Study. J Pediatr 2007; 150(1):12-7.e2. PMID: 17188605

32. Goldhaber-Fiebert JD, Rubinfeld RE, Bhattacharya J, Robinson TN, Wise PH. The Utility of Childhood and Adolescent Obesity Assessment in Relation to Adult Health. Med Decis Making 2012. PMID: 22647830

33. Reilly JJ, Kelly J. Long-term impact of overweight and obesity in childhood and adolescence on morbidity and premature mortality in adulthood: systematic review. Int J Obes (Lond) 2010. PMID: 20975725

34. Li L, Pinot de Moira A, Power C. Predicting cardiovascular disease risk factors in midadulthood from childhood body mass index: utility of different cutoffs for childhood BMI. Am J Clin Nutr 2011. PMID: 21430113

35. Wang Y, Beydoun MA, Liang L, Caballero B, Kumanyika SK. Will all Americans become overweight or obese? estimating the progression and cost of the US obesity epidemic. Obesity (Silver Spring) 2008; 16(10):2323-30. PMID: 18719634

36. Thomson Medstat Research Brief: Childhood Obesity: Costs, Treatment Patterns, Disparities in Care and Prevalent Medical Conditions, 2006, found at: http://www.medstat.com/pdfs/childhood_obesity.pdf .

37. Hampl SE, Carroll CA, Simon SD, et al. Resource utilization and expenditures for overweight and obese children. Arch. Pediatr. Adolesc. Med. 2007; 161(1):11-4. PMID: 17199061.

38. Hampl SE, Summar MJ. 'Weighing in' on childhood obesity. Pediatr Ann. 2009 March;38(3):143-8. PMID: 19353903.

39. Bray JA, James WPT, Bouchard C. Handbook Of Obesity, Second Edition. New York: Marcel Dekker, INC, 1998.

40. Whitlock EP, O'Connor EA, Williams SB, Beil TL, Lutz KW. Effectiveness of weight management interventions in children: a targeted systematic review for the USPSTF. Pediatrics 2010; 125(2):e396-418. PMID: 20083531

41. Moher D, Liberati A, Tetzlaff J, Altman DG. Preferred reporting items for systematic reviews and meta-analyses: the PRISMA statement. BMJ 2009; 339:b2535. PMID: 19622551

42. Human Development Reports. Human Development Index. http://hdr.undp.org/en/statistics/hdi/. Last accessed 21 May 2012.

43. Downs SH, Black N. The feasibility of creating a checklist for the assessment of the methodological quality both of randomised and non-randomised studies of health care interventions. J Epidemiol Community Health 1998; 52(6):377-84. PMID: 9764259

44. DerSimonian R, Laird N. Meta-analysis in clinical trials. Control Clin Trials. 1986 Sept;7(3):177-88. PMID: 3802833.

45. Donnelly JE, Greene JL, Gibson CA et al. Physical Activity Across the Curriculum (PAAC): a randomized controlled trial to promote physical activity and diminish overweight and obesity in elementary school children. Prev Med 2009; 49(4):336-41. PMID: 19665037

46. Foster GD, Linder B, Baranowski T et al. A school-based intervention for diabetes risk reduction. N Engl J Med. 2010 July 29;363(5):443-53. PMID: 20581420.

47. Graf C, Koch B, Falkowski G et al. School-based prevention: effects on obesity and physical performance after 4 years. J Sports Sci 2008; 26(10):987-94. PMID: 18608843

48. Gutin B, Yin Z, Johnson M, Barbeau P. Preliminary findings of the effect of a 3-year after-school physical activity intervention on fitness and body fat: the Medical College of Georgia Fitkid Project. Int J Pediatr Obes 2008; 3 Suppl 1:3-9. PMID: 18278626

49. James J, Thomas P, Cavan D, Kerr D. Preventing childhood obesity by reducing consumption of carbonated drinks: Cluster randomised controlled trial. Br. Med. J. 2004; 328(7450):1237-9. PMID: 15107313.

50. Neumark-Sztainer DR, Friend SE, Flattum CF et al. New moves-preventing weight-related problems in adolescent girls a group-randomized study. Am J Prev Med 2010; 39(5):421-32. PMID: 20965379

51. Sahota P, Rudolf MC, Dixey R, Hill AJ, Barth JH, Cade J. Randomised controlled trial of primary school based intervention to reduce risk factors for obesity. BMJ 2001; 323(7320):1029-32. PMID: 11691759

52. Walther C, Gaede L, Adams V et al. Effect of increased exercise in school children on physical fitness and endothelial progenitor cells: a prospective randomized trial. Circulation 2009; 120(22):2251-9. PMID: 19920000

53. Warren JM, Henry CJ, Lightowler HJ, Bradshaw SM, Perwaiz S. Evaluation of a pilot school programme aimed at the prevention of obesity in children. Health Promot Int 2003; 18(4):287-96. PMID: 14695360

54. James J, Thomas P, Kerr D. Preventing childhood obesity: Two year follow-up results from the Christchurch obesity prevention programme in schools (CHOPPS). BMJ: British Medical Journal. 2007; 335(7623):1-6. PMID: 17923721.

55. Muckelbauer R, Libuda L, Clausen K, Toschke AM, Reinehr T, Kersting M. Promotion and provision of drinking water in schools for overweight prevention: randomized, controlled cluster trial. Pediatrics 2009; 123(4):e661-7. PMID: 19336356

56. Gortmaker SL, Peterson K, Wiecha J et al. Reducing obesity via a school-based interdisciplinary intervention among youth: Planet Health. Arch Pediatr Adolesc Med 1999; 153(4):409-18. PMID: 10201726

57. Howe C, Harris R, Gutin B. A 10-month physical activity intervention improves body composition in young black boys. Journal of Obesity 2011; 8p. PMID: 20981151.

58. Llargues E, Recasens A, Franco R et al. Medium-term evaluation of an educational intervention on dietary and physical exercise habits in schoolchildren: The Avall 2 study: Evaluacion a medio plazo de una intervencion educativa en habitos alimentarios y de actividad fisica en escolares: Estudio Avall 2. Endocrinol Nutr. 2012; 59(5):288-95. PMID: 22521298.

59. Lubans DR, Morgan PJ, Callister R. Potential moderators and mediators of intervention effects in an obesity prevention program for adolescent boys from disadvantaged schools. J Sci Med Sport 2012. PMID: 22575499.

60. Lubans DR, Morgan PJ, Okely AD et al. Preventing Obesity Among Adolescent Girls: One-Year Outcomes of the Nutrition and Enjoyable Activity for Teen Girls (NEAT Girls) Cluster Randomized Controlled Trial. Arch Pediatr Adolesc Med 2012. PMID: 22566517

61. Magnusson KT, Hrafnkelsson H, Sigurgeirsson I, Johannsson E, Sveinsson T. Limited effects of a 2-year school-based physical activity intervention on body composition and cardiorespiratory fitness in 7-year-old children. Health Education Research 2012; 27(3):484-94. PMID: 22456632.

62. Rosario R, Oliveira B, Araujo A et al. The impact of an intervention taught by trained teachers on childhood overweight. Int. J. Environ. Res. Public Health 2012; 9(4):1355-67. PMID: 22690198.

63. Rush E, Reed P, McLennan S, et al.. A school-based obesity control programme: Project Energize. Two-year outcomes. British Journal of Nutrition. 2012; 107(4):581-7. PMID: 21733268.

64. Coleman KJ, Shordon M, Caparosa SL, et al. Changing nutrition policies and environments in low-income schools using implementation models: The healthy options for nutrition environments in schools (ONES) intervention. Obesity. 2011; 19:S124. http://www.embase.com/search/results?subaction=viewrecord&from=export&id=L70680833

65. DeBar LL, Schneider M, Drews KL et al. Student public commitment in a school-based diabetes prevention project: impact on physical health and health behavior. BMC Public Health 2011; 11:711.

66. Walter HJ, Hofman A, Connelly PA, Barrett LT, Kost KL. Primary prevention of chronic disease in childhood: changes in risk factors after one year of intervention. Am J Epidemiol 1985; 122(5):772-81. PMID: 4050769

67. Madsen J, Sallis JF, Rupp JW et al. Relationship between self-monitoring of diet and exercise change and subsequent risk factor changes in children and adults. Patient Educ Couns. 1993; 21(1-2):61-9. PMID: 8337206.

68. Barbeau P, Johnson MH, Howe CA et al. Ten months of exercise improves general and visceral adiposity, bone, and fitness in black girls. Obesity (Silver Spring) 2007; 15(8):2077-85. PMID: 17712126

69. Treviño RP, Hernandez AE, Yin Z, Garcia OA, Hernandez I. Effect of the Bienestar Health Program on Physical Fitness in Low-Income Mexican American Children. Hispanic Journal of Behavioral Sciences 2005; 27(1):120-32. http://search.ebscohost.com/login.aspx?direct=true&db=psyh&AN=2005-01342-007&site=ehost-live.

70. Bush PJ, Zuckerman AE, Theiss PK et al. Cardiovascular risk factor prevention in black schoolchildren: two-year results of the "Know Your Body" program. Am J Epidemiol 1989; 129(3):466-82. PMID: 2916540

71. Haerens L, Deforche B, Maes L, Stevens V, Cardon G, De Bourdeaudhuij I. Body mass effects of a physical activity and healthy food intervention in middle schools. Obesity (Silver Spring) 2006; 14(5):847-54. PMID: 16855194

72. Amaro S, Di Costanzo A, Madeo I et al. Kaledo, a new educational board-game, gives nutritional rudiments and encourages healthy eating in children: A pilot cluster randomized trial. European Journal of Pediatrics 2006; 165(9):630-5. PMID: 16733670.

73. Martínez Vizcaíno V, Salcedo Aguilar F, Franquelo Gutiérrez R et al. Assessment of an after-school physical activity program to prevent obesity among 9- to 10-year-old children: a cluster randomized trial. International Journal of Obesity (2005) 2008; 32(1):12-22. PMID: 17895883.

74. Klish WJ, Karavias KE, White KS et al. Multicomponent school-initiated obesity intervention in a high-risk, Hispanic elementary school. J. Pediatr Gastroenterol Nutr. 2012; 54(1):113-6. PMID: 21857252.

75. Sallis JF, McKenzie TL, Conway TL et al. Environmental interventions for eating and physical activity: a randomized controlled trial in middle schools. Am J Prev Med 2003; 24(3):209-17. PMID: 12657338

76. Thivel D, Isacco L, Lazaar N et al. Effect of a 6-month school-based physical activity program on body composition and physical fitness in lean and obese schoolchildren. Eur J Pediatr. 2011; 1-9. PMID: 21475968.

77. Metcalf B, Wilkin T, Puder J, et al. Lifestyle intervention has little effect on obesity. Comment on Puder JJ, Marques-Vidal P, Schindler C, , et al. Effect of multidimensional lifestyle intervention on fitness and adiposity in predominantly migrant preschool children (Ballabeina): cluster randomised controlled trial. BMJ 2011;343:d6195. (13 October.). BMJ: British Medical Journal (Overseas & Retired Doctors Edition) 2012; 344(7842):32-3. PMID: 22293374.

78 Kafatos A, Manios Y, Moschandreas J et al. Health and nutrition education in primary schools of Crete: Follow-up changes in body mass index and overweight status. Eur. J. Clin. Nutr. 2005; 59(9):1090-2. PMID: 16015265.

79. Lazaar N, Aucouturier J, Ratel S, Rance M, Meyer M, Duche P. Effect of physical activity intervention on body composition in young children: Influence of body mass index status and gender. Acta Paediatr. Int. J. Paediatr. 2007; 96(9):1315-20. PMID: 17718785.

80. Salmon J, Ball K, Hume C, Booth M, Crawford D. Outcomes of a group-randomized trial to prevent excess weight gain, reduce screen behaviours and promote physical activity in 10-year-old children: switch-play. Int J Obes (Lond) 2008; 32(4):601-12. PMID: 18253162

81. Jago R, McMurray RG, Drews KL et al. HEALTHY Intervention: Fitness, Physical Activity and Metabolic Syndrome Results. Med Sci Sports Exerc 2011. PMID: 21233778

82. Reed KE, Warburton DE, Macdonald HM, et al. Action Schools! BC: a school-based physical activity intervention designed to decrease cardiovascular disease risk factors in children. Preventive Medicine. 2008; 46(6):525-31. PMID: 18377970.

83. Vandongen R, Jenner DA, Thompson C et al. A controlled evaluation of a fitness and nutrition intervention program on cardiovascular health in 10- to 12-year-old children. Prev Med 1995; 24(1):9-22. PMID: 7740021

84. Kain J, Leyton B, Cerda R, et al. Two-year controlled effectiveness trial of a school-based intervention to prevent obesity in Chilean children. Public Health Nutr. 2009; 12(9):1451-61. PMID: 19102808.

85. Newton RL Jr, Han H, Anton SD et al. An environmental intervention to prevent excess weight gain in African-American students: a pilot study. Am J Health Promot 2010; 24(5):340-3. PMID: 20465148

86. Sallis JF, McKenzie TL, Alcaraz JE, et al. Project SPARK. Effects of physical education on adiposity in children. Ann New York Acad Sci. 1993; 699:127-36. PMID: 8267303.

87. Resaland GK, Anderssen SA, Holme IM, Mamen A, Andersen LB. Effects of a 2-year school-based daily physical activity intervention on cardiovascular disease risk factors: the Sogndal school-intervention study. Scandinavian Journal of Medicine & Science in Sports. 2011; 21(6):e122-31. PMID: 22126720.

88. Stock S, Miranda C, Evans S, et al. Healthy buddies: A novel, peer-led health promotion program for the prevention of obesity and eating disorders in children in elementary school. Pediatrics. 2007; 120(4):e1059-e1068. PMID: 17908726.

89. Smolak L, Levine MP. A two-year follow-up of a primary prevention program for negative body image and unhealthy weight regulation. Eating Disord. 2001; 9(4):313-25. PMID: 16864392.

90. Fung C, Kuhle S, Lu C et al. From "best practice" to "next practice": The effectiveness of school-based health promotion in improving healthy eating and physical activity and preventing childhood obesity. 2012;27. PMID: 22413778.

91. Burguera B, Colom A, Pinero E et al. ACTYBOSS: Activity, behavioral therapy in young subjects - After-school intervention pilot project on obesity prevention. Obes Facts. 2011; 4(5):400-6. PMID: 22166761.

92. Stenevi-Lundgren S, Daly RM, Linden C, Gardsell P, Karlsson MK. Effects of a daily school based physical activity intervention program on muscle development in prepubertal girls. Eur J Appl Physiol. 2009; 105(4):533-41. PMID: 19018558.

93. Viskic-Stalec N, Stalec J, Katic R, Podvorac D, Katovic D. The impact of dance-aerobics training on the morpho-motor status in female high-schoolers. Coll Antropol 2007; 31(1):259-66. PMID: 17598411

94. Damon S, Dietrich S, Widhalm K. PRESTO - Prevention Study of Obesity: A project to prevent obesity during childhood and adolescence. Acta Paediatr Int J Paediatr. 2005; 94(SUPP. 448):47-8. PMID: 16175809.

95. Heelan KA, Abbey BM, Donnelly JE, Mayo MS, Welk GJ. Evaluation of a walking school bus for promoting physical activity in youth. J Phys Act Health 2009; 6(5):560-7. PMID: 19953832

96. Skybo TA, Ryan-Wenger N. A school-based intervention to teach third grade children about the prevention of heart disease. Pediatr Nurs 2002; 28(3):223-9, 235. PMID: 12087641

97. Tucker S, Lanningham-Foster L, Murphy J et al. A school based community partnership for promoting healthy habits for life. J Community Health 2011; 36(3):414-22. PMID: 20976532

98. Sollerhed A-C, Ejlertsson G. Physical benefits of expanded physical education in primary school: Findings from a 3-year intervention study in Sweden. Scandinavian Journal of Medicine & Science in Sports 2008; 18(1):102-7. PMID: 17490464.

99. Taylor RW, McAuley KA, Barbezat W, Strong A, Williams SM, Mann JI. APPLE Project: 2-y findings of a community-based obesity prevention program in primary school age children. Am J Clin Nutr 2007; 86(3):735-42. PMID: 17823440

100. Manios Y, Kafatos A. Health and nutrition education in primary schools in Crete: 10 years follow-up of serum lipids, physical activity and macronutrient intake. Br J Nutr 2006; 95(3):568-75. PMID: 16578934

101. Valdimarsson O, Linden C, Johnell O, Gardsell P, Karlsson MK. Daily physical education in the school curriculum in prepubertal girls during 1 year is followed by an increase in bone mineral accrual and bone width--data from the prospective controlled Malmö pediatric osteoporosis prevention study. Calcified Tissue International 2006; 78(2):65-71.

102. Scheffler C, Ketelhut K, Mohasseb I. Does physical education modify the body composition?--results of a longitudinal study of pre-school children. Anthropol Anz 2007; 65(2):193-201. PMID: 17711151

103. Manios Y, Moschandreas J, Hatzis C, Kafatos A. Evaluation of a health and nutrition education program in primary school children of Crete over a three-year period. Prev Med 1999; 28(2):149-59. PMID: 10048106

104. Manios Y, Moschandreas J, Hatzis C, et al. Health and nutrition education in primary schools of Crete: Changes in chronic disease risk factors following a 6-year intervention programme. British Journal of Nutrition 2002; 88(3):315-24. PMID: 12207842.

105. Bronikowski M, Bronikowska M. Will they stay fit and healthy? A three-year follow-up evaluation of a physical activity and health intervention in Polish youth. Scandinavian Journal of Public Health 2011; 39(7):704-13. PMID: 21948996.

106. Chiodera P, Volta E, Gobbi G et al. Specifically designed physical exercise programs improve children's motor abilities. Scandinavian Journal of Medicine & Science in Sports. 2008; 18(2):179-87. PMID: 17490452.

107. McArthur L, Holbert D, Pena M. Obesity knowledge of adolescents from six Latin American cities: A multivariable analysis. Nutr. Res. 2001 July; 21(10):1323-33.http://www.embase.com/search/results?subaction=viewrecord&from=export&id=L34024012

108. Salcedo Aguilar F, Martínez-Vizcaíno V, Sánchez López M et al. Impact of an after-school physical activity program on obesity in children. The Journal of Pediatrics 2010; 157(1):36-42.e3. PMID: 20227726.

109. Brey RL, Stallworth CL, McGlasson DL et al. Antiphospholipid antibodies and stroke in young women. Stroke 2002; 33(10):2396-400. PMID: 12364727

110. Yin Z, Gutin B, Johnson MH et al. An environmental approach to obesity prevention in children: Medical College of Georgia FitKid Project year 1 results. Obes Res 2005; 13(12):2153-61. PMID: 16421350

111. Slykerman RF, Thompson JMD, Pryor JE et al. Maternal stress, social support and preschool children's intelligence. Early Hum. Dev. 2005; 81(10):815-21. PMID: 16019165.

112. Will JC, Massoudi B, Mokdad A et al. Reducing risk for cardiovascular disease in uninsured women: combined results from two WISEWOMAN projects. Journal of the American Medical Women's Association (1972) 2001; 56(4):161-5. PMID: 11759784.

113. Worthmann H, Schwartz A, Heidenreich F et al. Educational campaign on stroke in an urban population in Northern Germany: influence on public stroke awareness and knowledge. Int J Stroke 2012. PMID: 22568388

114. Trevino RP, Yin Z, Hernandez A, Hale DE, Garcia OA, Mobley C. Impact of the Bienestar school-based diabetes mellitus prevention program on fasting capillary glucose levels: a randomized controlled trial. Arch Pediatr Adolesc Med 2004; 158(9):911-7. PMID: 15351759

115. Caballero B, Clay T, Davis SM et al. Pathways: a school-based, randomized controlled trial for the prevention of obesity in American Indian schoolchildren. Am J Clin Nutr 2003; 78(5):1030-8. PMID: 14594792

116. Hendy HM, Williams KE, Camise TS. Kid's Choice Program improves weight management behaviors and weight status in school children. Appetite 2011; 56(2):484-94. PMID: 21277924

117. Robinson TN. Reducing children's television viewing to prevent obesity: a randomized controlled trial. JAMA 1999; 282(16):1561-7. PMID: 10546696

118. Burke V, Milligan RA, Thompson C et al. A controlled trial of health promotion programs in 11-year-olds using physical activity "enrichment" for higher risk children. J Pediatr 1998; 132(5):840-8. PMID: 9602197

119. Dzewaltowski DA, Rosenkranz RR, Geller KS et al. HOP'N after-school project: an obesity prevention randomized controlled trial. Int J Behav Nutr Phys Act 2010; 7:90. PMID: 21144055

120. Danielzik S, Pust S, Muller MJ. School-based interventions to prevent overweight and obesity in prepubertal children: Process and 4-years outcome evaluation of the Kiel Obesity Prevention Study (KOPS). Acta Paediatr. Int. J. Paediatr. 2007; 96(SUPPL. 454):19-25. PMID: 17313410.

121. Kriemler S, Zahner L, Schindler C et al. Effect of school based physical activity programme (KISS) on fitness and adiposity in primary schoolchildren: cluster randomised controlled trial. BMJ 2010; 340:c785. PMID: 20179126

122. Nader PR, Stone EJ, Lytle LA et al. Three-year maintenance of improved diet and physical activity: The CATCH cohort. Archives of Pediatrics & Adolescent Medicine 1999; 153(7):695-704. PMID: 10401802.

123. Mihas C, Mariolis A, Manios Y et al. Evaluation of a nutrition intervention in adolescents of an urban area in Greece: short- and long-term effects of the VYRONAS study. Public Health Nutr 2010; 13(5):712-9. PMID: 19781127

124. Hatzis CM, Papandreou C, Kafatos AG. School health education programs in Crete: Evaluation of behavioural and health indices a decade after initiation. Preventive Medicine: An International Journal Devoted to Practice and Theory 2010; 51(3-4):262-7. PMID: 20566355.

125. Marcus C, Nyberg G, Nordenfelt A, Karpmyr M, Kowalski J, Ekelund U. A 4-year, cluster-randomized, controlled childhood obesity prevention study: STOPP. Int J Obes (Lond) 2009; 33(4):408-17. PMID: 19290010

126. Story M, Hannan PJ, Fulkerson JA et al. Bright Start: Description and Main Outcomes From a Group-Randomized Obesity Prevention Trial in American Indian Children. Obesity 2012. PMID: 22513491.

127. Brandstetter S, Klenk J, Berg S et al. Overweight prevention implemented by primary school teachers: A randomised controlled trial. Obes Facts. 2012; 5(1):1-11. PMID: 22433612.

128. Llargues E, Franco R, Recasens A et al. Assessment of a school-based intervention in eating habits and physical activity in school children: the AVall study. Journal of Epidemiology & Community Health. 2011; 65(10):896-901. PMID: 21398682.

129. Lloyd JJ, Wyatt KM, Creanor S. Behavioural and weight status outcomes from an exploratory trial of the Healthy Lifestyles Programme (HeLP): a novel school-based obesity prevention programme. BMJ Open 2012; 2(3). PMID: 22586282

130. Williamson DA, Champagne CM, Harsha DW et al. Effect of an Environmental School-Based Obesity Prevention Program on Changes in Body Fat and Body Weight: A Randomized Trial. Obesity (Silver Spring) 2012. PMID: 22402733

131. Siegrist M, Lammel C, Haller B, Christle J, Halle M. Effects of a physical education program on physical activity, fitness, and health in children: The JuvenTUM project. Scand J Med Sci Sports 2011. PMID: 22092492

132. Simon C, Schweitzer B, Oujaa M et al. Successful overweight prevention in adolescents by increasing physical activity: a 4-year randomized controlled intervention. Int J Obes (Lond) 2008; 32(10):1489-98. PMID: 18626482

133. Foster GD, Sherman S, Borradaile KE et al. A policy-based school intervention to prevent overweight and obesity. Pediatrics 2008; 121(4):e794-802. PMID: 18381508

134. Hopper CA, Munoz KD, Gruber MB, Nguyen KP. The effects of a family fitness program on the physical activity and nutrition behaviors of third-grade children. Res Q Exerc Sport 2005; 76(2):130-9. PMID: 16128481

135. Manios Y, Kafatos A, Mamalakis G. The effects of a health education intervention initiated at first grade over a 3 year period: physical activity and fitness indices. Health Educ Res 1998; 13(4):593-606. PMID: 10345909

136. Shofan Y, Kedar O, Branski D, et al. A school-based program of physical activity may prevent obesity. Eur J Clin Nutr. 2011; 65(6):768-70. PMID: 21427748.

137. Simonetti D'Arca A, Tarsitani G, Cairella M. Prevention of obesity in elementary and nursery school children. Public Health. 1986; 100(3):166-73. PMID: 3737864.

138. Hollar D, Messiah SE, Lopez-Mitnik G, Hollar TL, Almon M, Agatston AS. Effect of a two-year obesity prevention intervention on percentile changes in body mass index and academic performance in low-income elementary school children. Am J Public Health 2010; 100(4):646-53. PMID: 20167892

139. Hoelscher DM, Springer AE, Ranjit N et al. Reductions in child obesity among disadvantaged school children with community involvement: the Travis County CATCH Trial. Obesity (Silver Spring) 2010; 18 Suppl 1:S36-44. PMID: 20107459

140. Lionis C, Kafatos A, Vlachonikolis J, et al. The effects of a health education intervention program among Cretan adolescents. Preventive Medicine. 1991; 20:685-99. PMID: 1766941.

141. Schetzina KE, Dalton WT 3rd, Lowe EF et al. A coordinated school health approach to obesity prevention among Appalachian youth: the Winning with Wellness Pilot Project. Fam Community Health 2009; 32(3):271-85. PMID: 19525708

142. Speroni KG, Earley C, Atherton M. Evaluating the effectiveness of the Kids Living Fit program: a comparative study. J Sch Nurs 2007; 23(6):329-36. PMID: 18052518

143. Coleman KJ, Tiller CL, Sanchez J et al. Prevention of the epidemic increase in child risk of overweight in low-income schools: the El Paso coordinated approach to child health. Arch Pediatr Adolesc Med 2005; 159(3):217-24. PMID: 15753263

144. Gorely T, Nevill ME, Morris JG, Stensel DJ, Nevill A. Effect of a school-based intervention to promote healthy lifestyles in 7-11 year old children. Int J Behav Nutr Phys Act 2009; 6:5. PMID: 19154622

145. Tseng M, Olufade TO, Evers KA, et al. Adolescent lifestyle factors and adult breast density in U.S. Chinese immigrant women. Nutrition & Cancer. 2011; 63(3):342-9. PMID: 21391125.

146. Angelopoulos PD, Milionis HJ, Grammatikaki E, Moschonis G, Manios Y. Changes in BMI and blood pressure after a school based intervention: the CHILDREN study. Eur J Public Health 2009; 19(3):319-25. PMID: 19208697

147. Greening L, Harrell KT, Low AK, Fielder CE. Efficacy of a school-based childhood obesity intervention program in a rural southern community: TEAM Mississippi Project. Obesity (Silver Spring) 2011; 19(6):1213-9. PMID: 21233806

148. Jansen W, Borsboom G, Meima A et al. Effectiveness of a primary school-based intervention to reduce overweight. Int J Pediatr Obes. 2011; 6(2 -2):e70-e77. PMID: 21609245.

149. De Coen V, De Bourdeaudhuij I, Vereecken C et al. Effects of a 2-year healthy eating and physical activity intervention for 3-6-year-olds in communities of high and low socio-economic status: the POP (Prevention of Overweight among Pre-school and school children) project. Public Health Nutr 2012; 1-9. PMID: 22397833

150. de Meij JS, Chinapaw MJ, van Stralen MM, van der Wal MF, van Dieren L, van Mechelen W. Effectiveness of JUMP-in, a Dutch primary school-based community intervention aimed at the promotion of physical activity. Br J Sports Med 2010. PMID: 21112875

151. Sanigorski AM, Bell AC, Kremer PJ, Cuttler R, Swinburn BA. Reducing unhealthy weight gain in children through community capacity-building: results of a quasi-experimental intervention program, Be Active Eat Well. Int J Obes (Lond) 2008; 32(7):1060-7. PMID: 18542082

152. Millar L, Kremer P, de Silva-Sanigorski A et al. Reduction in overweight and obesity from a 3-year community-based intervention in Australia: the 'It's Your Move!' project. Obes Rev 2011; 12 Suppl 2:20-8. PMID: 22008556

153. Naul R, Schmelt D, Dreiskaemper D, Hoffmann D, l'Hoir M. 'Healthy children in sound communities' (HCSC/gkgk)--a Dutch-German community-based network project to counteract obesity and physical inactivity. Fam Pract 2012; 29 Suppl 1:i110-i116. PMID: 22399539

154. Tomlin D, Naylor PJ, McKay H, Zorzi A, Mitchell M, Panagiotopoulos C. The impact of Action Schools! BC on the health of Aboriginal children and youth living in rural and remote communities in British Columbia. Int J Circumpolar Health 2012; 71:17999. PMID: 22456048

155. Johnson BA, Kremer PJ, Swinburn BA, de Silva-Sanigorski AM. Multilevel analysis of the Be Active Eat Well intervention: environmental and behavioural influences on reductions in child obesity risk. Int J Obes. 2012. PMID: 22531087.

156. Kazemi M, Rahman A, De Ciantis M. Weight cycling in adolescent Taekwondo athletes. Journal of the Canadian Chiropractic Association. 2011;55(4):318-24. PMID: 22131569.

157. Swami V, Tovee MJ. Big beautiful women: the body size preferences of male fat admirers. J Sex Res 2009; 46(1):89-96. PMID: 19116865

158. Muckelbauer R, Libuda L, Clausen K, Reinehr T, Kersting M. A simple dietary intervention in the school setting decreased incidence of overweight in children. Obes Facts 2009; 2(5):282-5. PMID: 20057194

159. Webber LS, Catellier DJ, Lytle LA et al. Promoting physical activity in middle school girls: Trial of Activity for Adolescent Girls. Am J Prev Med 2008; 34(3):173-84. PMID: 18312804

160. Crespo NC, Elder JP, Ayala GX et al. Results of a multi-level intervention to prevent and control childhood obesity among Latino children: the Aventuras Para Ninos Study. Ann Behav Med 2012; 43(1):84-100. PMID: 22215470

161. Macaulay AC, Paradis G, Potvin L et al. The Kahnawake Schools Diabetes Prevention Project: intervention, evaluation, and baseline results of a diabetes primary prevention program with a native community in Canada. Prev Med 1997; 26(6):779-90. PMID: 9388789

162. Madsen KA, Thompson HR, Wlasiuk L, et al. After-school program to reduce obesity in minority children: A pilot study. Journal of Child Health Care 2009; 13(4):333-46. PMID: 19833672.

163. Utter J, Scragg R, Robinson E et al. Evaluation of the Living 4 Life project: A youth-led, school-based obesity prevention study. Obes Rev 2011; 12(SUPPL. 2):51-60. PMID: 22008559.

164. Muckelbauer R, Libuda L, Clausen K, Toschke AM, Reinehr T, Kersting M. Immigrational background affects the effectiveness of a school-based overweight prevention program promoting water consumption. Obesity (Silver Spring) 2010; 18(3):528-34. PMID: 19713953

165. Schneider M, Dunton GF, Bassin S, Graham DJ, Eliakim A, Cooper DM. impact of a school-based physical activity intervention on fitness and bone in adolescent females. Journal of Physical Activity & Health. 2007; 4(1):17-29. PMID: 17489004.

166. Spiegel SA, Foulk D. Reducing overweight through a multidisciplinary school-based intervention. Obesity (Silver Spring, Md.). 2006; 14(1):88-96. PMID: 16493126.

167. Prins RG, Brug J, van Empelen P, Oenema A. Effectiveness of YouRAction, an intervention to promote adolescent physical activity using personal and environmental feedback: A cluster RCT. PLoS ONE 2012; 7(3). PMID: 22403695.

168. Ezendam NPM, Brug J, Oenema A. Evaluation of the web-based computer-tailored FATaintPHAT intervention to promote energy balance among adolescents: Results from a school cluster randomized trial. Arch Pediatr Adolesc Med. 2012; 166(3):248-55. PMID: 22064878.

169. Kómár M, Nagymajté nyi L, Nyári T, et al. The determinants of self-rated health among ethnic minorities in Hungary. Ethnicity & Health 2006; 11(2):121-32. PMID: 16595315.

170. Gorely T, Morris JG, Musson H, et al. Physical activity and body composition outcomes of the GreatFun2Run intervention at 20 month follow-up. International Journal of Behavioral Nutrition & Physical Activity. 2011; 8:11p. PMID: 21767356.

171. Epstein LH, Gordy CC, Raynor HA, Beddome M, Kilanowski CK, Paluch R. Increasing fruit and vegetable intake and decreasing fat and sugar intake in families at risk for childhood obesity. Obes Res 2001; 9(3):171-8. PMID: 11323442

172. Lappe JM, Rafferty KA, Davies KM, Lypaczewski G. Girls on a high-calcium diet gain weight at the same rate as girls on a normal diet: a pilot study. J Am Diet Assoc 2004; 104(9):1361-7. PMID: 15354150

173. French SA, Gerlach AF, Mitchell NR, et al. Household obesity prevention: Take action-a group-randomized trial. Obesity. 2011; 19(10):2082-8. PMID: 23404749.

174. Fitzgibbon ML, Stolley MR, Schiffer L et al. Family-Based Hip-Hop to Health: Outcome Results. Obesity (Silver Spring) 2012. PMID: 22644499

175. Patrick K, Calfas KJ, Norman GJ et al. Randomized controlled trial of a primary care and home-based intervention for physical activity and nutrition behaviors: PACE+ for adolescents. Arch Pediatr Adolesc Med 2006; 160(2):128-36. PMID: 16461867

176. Gentile DA, Welk G, Eisenmann JC et al. Evaluation of a multiple ecological level child obesity prevention program: Switch what you Do, View, and Chew. BMC Med 2009; 7:49. PMID: 19765270

177. Polacsek M, Orr J, Letourneau L et al. Impact of a primary care intervention on physician practice and patient and family behavior: Keep ME Healthy--The Maine Youth Overweight Collaborative. Pediatrics 2009; 123(Suppl):258-66. PMID: 19470601.

178. Tanofsky-Kraff M, Wilfley DE, Young JF, et al. A pilot study of interpersonal psychotherapy for preventing excess weight gain in adolescent girls at-risk for obesity. Int J Eating Disord. 2010; 43(8):701-6. PMID: 19882739.

179. Bayer O, von Kries R, Strauss A et al. Short- and mid-term effects of a setting based prevention program to reduce obesity risk factors in children: a cluster-randomized trial. Clin Nutr 2009; 28(2):122-8. PMID: 19303675

180. Fitzgibbon ML, Stolley MR, Schiffer L, Van Horn L, KauferChristoffel K, Dyer A. Hip-Hop to Health Jr. for Latino preschool children Obesity (Silver Spring) 2006; 14(9):1616-25. PMID: 17030973

181. Burgi F, Niederer I, Schindler C et al. Effect of a lifestyle intervention on adiposity and fitness in socially disadvantaged subgroups of preschoolers: A cluster-randomized trial (Ballabeina). Prev Med. 2012; 54(5):335-40. PMID: 22373886.

182. Eiholzer U, Meinhardt U, Petro R, Witassek F, Gutzwiller F, Gasser T. High-intensity training increases spontaneous physical activity in children: a randomized controlled study. J Pediatr 2010; 156(2):242-6. PMID: 19846114

183. Singh AS, Chin A Paw MJ, Brug J, van Mechelen W. Dutch obesity intervention in teenagers: effectiveness of a school-based program on body composition and behavior. Arch Pediatr Adolesc Med 2009; 163(4):309-17. PMID: 19349559

184. Chomitz VR, McGowan RJ, Wendel JM et al. Healthy Living Cambridge Kids: a community-based participatory effort to promote healthy weight and fitness. Obesity (Silver Spring) 2010; 18 Suppl 1:S45-53. PMID: 20107461

185. Economos CD, Hyatt RR, Goldberg JP et al. A community intervention reduces BMI z-score in children: Shape Up Somerville first year results. Obesity (Silver Spring) 2007; 15(5):1325-36. PMID: 17495210

186. Robinson TN, Matheson DM, Kraemer HC et al. A randomized controlled trial of culturally tailored dance and reducing screen time to prevent weight gain in low-income African American girls: Stanford GEMS. Arch Pediatr Adolesc Med 2010; 164(11):995-1004. PMID: 21041592

187. Klesges RC, Obarzanek E, Kumanyika S et al. The Memphis Girls' health Enrichment Multi-site Studies (GEMS): an evaluation of the efficacy of a 2-year obesity prevention program in African American girls. Arch Pediatr Adolesc Med 2010; 164(11):1007-14. PMID: 21041593

188. de Silva-Sanigorski AM, Bell AC, Kremer P et al. Reducing obesity in early childhood: results from Romp & Chomp, an Australian community-wide intervention program. Am J Clin Nutr 2010; 91(4):831-40. PMID: 20147472

189. Chang DI, Gertel-Rosenberg A, Drayton VL, Schmidt S, Angalet GB. A statewide strategy to battle child obesity in Delaware. Health Aff (Millwood) 2010; 29(3):481-90. PMID: 20194990

190. Resnicow K. School-based obesity prevention. Population versus high-risk interventions. ANN. NEW YORK ACAD. SCI. 1993; 699:154-66. PMID: http://www.embase.com/search/results?subaction=viewrecord&from=export&id=L23359976

191. Waters E, de Silva-Sanigorski A, Hall BJ et al. Interventions for preventing obesity in children. Cochrane Database Syst Rev 2011; (12):CD001871. PMID: 22161367

192. Institute of Medicine. (2012). Accelerating Progress in Obesity Prevention: Solving the Weight of the Nation. Washington, DC: National Academies Press. www.iom.edu/Reports/2012/Accelerating-Progress-in-Obesity-Prevention.aspx.

193. Hill JO, Wyatt HR, Reed GW, Peters JC. Obesity and the environment: where do we go from here? Science 2003; 299(5608):853-5. PMID: 12574618

194. Latner JD, Stunkard AJ. Getting worse: the stigmatization of obese children. Obes Res. 2003 Mar;11(3):452-6. PMID: 12634444.

195. Carter FA, Bulik CM. Childhood obesity prevention programs: how do they affect eating pathology and other psychological measures? Psychosom Med 2008; 70(3):363-71. PMID: 18378876

196. Berg F, Buechner J, Parham E. Guidelines for childhood obesity prevention programs: promoting healthy weight in children. J Nutr Educ Behav 2003; 35(1):1-4. PMID: 12596730

197. Zwiauer KF. Prevention and treatment of overweight and obesity in children and adolescents. Eur J Pediatr 2000; 159 Suppl 1:S56-68. PMID: 11011956

198. Kropski JA, Keckley PH, Jensen GL. School-based obesity prevention programs: an evidence-based review. Obesity (Silver Spring) 2008; 16(5):1009-18. PMID: 18356849

199. Jaime PC, Lock K. Do school based food and nutrition policies improve diet and reduce obesity? (Structured abstract). Preventive Medicine. 2009; 48(1):45-53. PMID: 19026676.

200. Doak CM, Visscher TL, Renders CM, Seidell JC. The prevention of overweight and obesity in children and adolescents: a review of interventions and programmes. Obes Rev 2006; 7(1):111-36. PMID: 16436107

201. Campbell K, Waters E, O'Meara S, Kelly S, Summerbell C. Interventions for preventing obesity in children. Cochrane Database Syst Rev 2002; (2):CD001871. PMID: 12076426

202. Kamath CC, Vickers KS, Ehrlich A et al. Clinical review: behavioral interventions to prevent childhood obesity: a systematic review and metaanalyses of randomized trials. J Clin Endocrinol Metab 2008; 93(12):4606-15. PMID: 18782880

203. Thomas H. Obesity prevention programs for children and youth: why are their results so modest? Health Educ Res 2006; 21(6):783-95. PMID: 17099075

204. Bautista-Castano I, Doreste J, Serra-Majem L. Effectiveness of interventions in the prevention of childhood obesity. Eur J Epidemiol 2004; 19(7):617-22. PMID: 15461192

205. Lopez-Dicastillo O, Grande G, Callery P. Parents' contrasting views on diet versus activity of children: Implications for health promotion and obesity prevention. Patient Education and Counseling 2010; 78(1):117-23. PMID: 19560306. olopezde@unav.es

206. Harris KC, Kuramoto LK, Schulzer M, Retallack JE. Effect of school-based physical activity interventions on body mass index in children: a meta-analysis. CMAJ 2009; 180(7):719-26. PMID: 19332753

207. Brennan L, Castro S, Brownson RC, Claus J, Orleans CT. Accelerating evidence reviews and broadening evidence standards to identify effective, promising, and emerging policy and environmental strategies for prevention of childhood obesity. Annu Rev Public Health 2011; 32:199-223. PMID: 21219169

174

208.   Institute of Medicine. (2010). Bridging the Evidence Gap in Obesity Prevention: A Framework to Inform Decision Making. Washington, DC: National Academies Press. www.iom.edu/Reports/2010/Bridging-the-Evidence-Gap-in-Obesity-Prevention-A-Framework-to-Inform-Decision-Making.aspx.